T0171626

Angels Talk

Jan Wilson

BALBOA.
PRESS
A DIVISION OF HAY HOUSE

Balboa Press books may be ordered through booksellers or by contacting:

Balboa Press
A Division of Hay House
1663 Liberty Drive
Bloomington, IN 47403
www.balboapress.com.au
1-(877) 407-4847

ISBN: 978-1-4525-0517-6 (sc)
ISBN: 978-1-4525-0518-3 (e)

Because of the dynamic nature of the Internet, any web addresses or links contained in this book may have changed since publication and may no longer be valid. The views expressed in this work are solely those of the author and do not necessarily reflect the views of the publisher, and the publisher hereby disclaims any responsibility for them.

The author of this book does not dispense medical advice or prescribe the use of any technique as a form of treatment for physical, emotional, or medical problems without the advice of a physician, either directly or indirectly. The intent of the author is only to offer information of a general nature to help you in your quest for emotional and spiritual well-being. In the event you use any of the information in this book for yourself, which is your constitutional right, the author and the publisher assume no responsibility for your actions.

Any people depicted in stock imagery provided by Thinkstock are models, and such images are being used for illustrative purposes only.
Certain stock imagery © Thinkstock.

Printed in the United States of America

Balboa Press rev. date: 10/25/2012

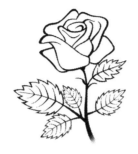

Angels Talk

As a rose is made by God, so are you.

A rose is a thing of beauty and joy

and this too, is your role in life.

You are like a rose:

from a bud to a perfect rose,

and then in age, still beautiful.

Mirror your life on a rose,

for it is showing you the way.

Serepis Bey

To Merlin and Maitreya
for guiding me while writing this special book for all to read.
With thanks to all the wonderful Ascended Masters
who have given their advice so that we may grow in knowledge.

To my dear husband Arty and all my family,
with love and thanks for being so wonderful
through my time of learning.

THE ASCENDED MASTERS ADVICE

THE REASON FOR THESE WRITINGS

1. To provide help for our angel helpers to bring in the New Age.
2. Why you are incarnated here at this time.
3. To show how to live a good life and enjoy it.
4. Why there is more awareness of the New Age.
5. So you are aware that the last lesson of your life is LOVE.
6. To show you the way to your Path of ascension.

These writings are a plea by the angels to all advanced souls to do your chosen job of helping the world improve and survive so that the promised New Age can be established. They are also written to help those of you in your last life, or lives, to find your Path of ascension to Heaven.

WHAT THE ANGELS SAID ABOUT THEIR WRITINGS.

MAITREYA 9/8/11
(a message for Jan)

Here is what is happening to you.

As you are writing, your words are those of a number of Ascended Masters and they have put their thoughts, based on their knowledge, through to you. Yes, this is who is speaking to you directly so that there can be no mistakes made. Our words are important and will help many people in their life.

Our words will not be prophecies of great deepness, but of ways for all to achieve the Light by finding their Path and to continue forward. We will also be showing how to provide the high vibrations that are necessary, so that God and His angels can fully bring in the New Age that is promised.

There are many seeking the right way and this we can achieve together.

Maitreya

INTRODUCTION

JAN'S STORY:

What happened to me was a truly an incredible experience!

While house sitting for some family members in January 2011, I found some daily inspirational cards and books available and these referred to different psychic abilities in which I had an interest. Each morning I used "The Ascended Masters Oracle Cards", by Doreen Virtue, which were thought provoking, and the random books I chose to look through enabled my mind to grasp some aspects that I had often wondered about. The main Oracle card that kept returning almost daily, was to write. I knew that this was a special moment in my life but I wondered about what I was to write and why I was receiving this idea.

On the 25th of January, 2011, I sat in my chair at home with a pen and paper and I heard a strong voice in my head. No name was given at this time, but the voice was firm and friendly and coming from behind my left ear. I started to write the words that I heard. Afterwards, I went to the Oracle cards and asked to be shown the name of the Master who spoke to me, and the card I was directed to was Merlin. The words I heard have formed Merlin's Prayer. He is the one who has led this first book of Life Truths along with the input of Maitreya and many other Ascended Masters. These many words that I've heard over the past year from 2011 to 2012, form a series of dissertations sent by the Ascended Masters for those of you who are looking for what life is about, and of how to handle all the situations that emerge in such a life as we have at this time. They are all provided by the Masters who give basic advice as to how to follow your own chosen Path. They show you ways to know when you are on the right Path or are being led astray by your negative ego. I have found this aspect of knowing the difference as vital to travelling my own Path!

These words were specifically directed and written for you, dear reader.

These stories are not mine! They were spoken through me as their medium, and as I heard the words, I wrote them. These Masters I know as my dear friends and their writings are lovingly presented for you and me. This book is written in the form of a "how to manual", so that all can access the information stored within. It is given with love from Heaven, and the writers, who by doing their chosen job of helping mankind, are giving freely to those of you who are seeking the information that you need to go forward in your personal journey of your Spirit's everlasting life. These Masters have now sent me their word that it is time to start sharing their writings, and so here you are. Those who are writing for this book include Jesus, Merlin, Maitreya, St.Germain and Serepis Bey, just to name a few you will know. I am told that one of the writings is from God Himself! There are writings from other Masters who may not be so well known to you, such as White Buffalo Calf Woman and Orchun, to name two, but their input is a wonderful help. Regardless of whether you know them or not, their writings are sent with love for all of you! Use this information well, for later when you want help, you will know how to reach your many angel helpers. You are never alone. You will know that help will be forth coming!

We are all God's children and these writings are to help us to master our life and our world so that we may enjoy the real pleasures that God intended to be in our life, and especially in this time of our last lives or our final life time prior to ascension.

These writings are also a plea from God and His angels to start the job that you undertook to do before you were born into this life. This commitment was to send positive vibrations to the angels so that they could then help the world in this negative situation that it finds itself in. Without you asking them, they cannot help the world and all in it. You always have the gift of free will and so the angels need your permission to help restore the world so that the New Age can replace that which is evil in this world today.

I will start with the first two writings I received, as this is what Merlin requested. Enjoy the words of Heaven, for they are simply stated and clearly written, with ideas you can follow or not, as your gift of free will takes you.

You will find that some statements and ideas will appear continuously throughout the writings, and these serve to remind you that these points should be kept to the forefront of your mind for these are important for you to know and use.

Take whatever comfort, love or lesson from what is written.

It is for you.

With love,
Jan

MERLIN 25/1/2011

As the world goes by, we shall be together.

We are One.

Together we shall win as One.

Be together, for togetherness is the Reality of Life.

Show me the way and all will be accomplished.

Find the answer to the Universe through our time together,

and spread it for all to know.

The Truth is such, that all shall be included in our knowledge.

The knowledge of the sea, and the earth, and the sky

will fill our minds,

and we are ready to do our work.
Amen

MERLIN 26/1/11

At the start we shall begin again.

Where do we begin?

At the beginning, of course,

And I say to you that all is good and calm, and we are together.

The learning begins.

As it was in the past, we shall be together.

Relax and enjoy, for all is good.

You are connected to me.

Many of us are on this journey with time and love to spend.

The world is moving forward rapidly. We shall assist it by divulging the Truth.

> The Truth is love for all.

> Amen.

MERLIN 27/1/11

I am your friend, and as one, we will seek to guide many.

We are the archangels and angels of Heaven and earth. We are here to help the people of earth adjust to the next part of the world's life. You have noticed that this is a tumultuous time in many countries, and this is not just due to unrest in the world, but because it is also growing and bringing in the new. Just as autumn does for spring, the world is clearing and cleansing for the new beginning.

The world will be an enlightened world full of love, faith and helping your fellow man. Despair not for those who appear to be suffering. In many minds they are, but others of you are aware that before your birth you chose a life that will help you develop spiritually. Each life you have is a part of growing and learning many lessons so that you can know your Spirit, which then takes you further on your journey. We will discuss this later. One can equate this life and each previous life as a kindergarten, then a primary school, and then high school. With what is a comparison of the higher education at an earthly University, in this advanced life you will start to become aware of the Secrets of Life and the joys that are available to all who seek the Light. Then, as University is a path to a degree, this heavenly education is the Path taking you in the direction of your ascension, for you are working through your final karma and ego driven responses. In this respect, the Path you are on is the way to your ascension. You are a blessed group as you are close to your ascension, and also helping the world into the New Age through the earliest days of this time. As God said, "The meek shall inherit the earth".

Some of you may study or go to metaphysical retreats, and others will read until they gain their own knowledge of what is occurring. This dear writer has not taken any courses but is an avid reader of all she can to find out about her journey. You are free to choose what you learn, but be aware that since you are reading this book, you have started your journey back Home to reside in the Light and to serve mankind. In what way will you serve, you ask? There are many ways. Look at your interests in this life and see if this interest is deep enough to continue. As there are uncountable jobs in the world, the same is valid in Heaven.

Your role is to serve and grow. Love will rule all.

As bad deeds that are done return as negative karma, good deeds will bring you advancement in your journey to the Light.

Blessings to you,
Merlin

LORD MAITREYA 21/5/11

Now to begin, I will tell you that you are going to learn about life as it is.

The problems of the world are being brought to notice due to the New Age which began before the start of the new millennium. Now, years later, people can see that there are cyclones, tornadoes, fires, earthquakes, tsunamis, and floods, as well as man induced trauma. These are present in a stronger form than has ever been seen before in the world's history. As Merlin has indicated, this is the world changing from the negative vibrations of the past age to the positive vibrations of this new one. We all realize that when a building is past its useful time, it is knocked down so that a better and more satisfactory structure can be built. This is what the natural disasters are achieving as well as the man-made disasters. Look at what happened in the Queensland floods which occurred at the beginning of January 2011 in Australia. After the event, many people from all over the country arrived to help freely with their tools, and their strength and a determination to help, for love of their fellow man. This is what we are now beginning to see, and this is how the future will be.

"Do unto others, as you would have them do unto you". Jesus shows the way to love, trust, and to have faith in other people of the world. Yes, it seems a severe way of turning people towards each other. When each of you are self sufficient and contented in your own space, there is not a lot of love outside of family and friends especially if it impinges on your self-satisfied state of ego, and more particularly, if the ones needing help are perceived as being "different". Certainly, money is given to help, but the real self is not often involved except for commenting on the tragedy of what is occurring. There is no real value or help in this attitude! This attitude is now slowly changing and people will be willing to give more of them self at a personal cost, not just a financial one. Citizens are now aware that they too may one day be involved in personal trauma and would then need to seek help from others. Do not be afraid of this world, for if you ask for your angels help, you will be cared for even if the problems seem insurmountable. Remember that you chose this life before you were born!

The future will be shining and new, but Now is all that is important for you. Live your life with the joy that is the Now of this time. The past has gone and the future has not arrived. There is only Now. Enjoy it! Enjoyment raises the vibrations of your body and the environment around you. You have all had an experience of divine joy. The memory remains because your body vibration was increased and lifted to the Light. The Light is where you come from and are seeking to return to and this place is called Heaven or Paradise. Your level of vibration will continue to rise up until after an inconceivable amount of births, lives and so called deaths, you will find yourself in your higher body of vibration and you will be ready for your last incarnation. As such, you will be on the Path to your ascension. Your training can be in schools or groups teaching about the Light, or in books such as this one. Once you are on the Path of becoming what is called "I Am Spirit", you will be guided to the knowledge that you require. You will be guided to certain areas of personal interest in which you can find your work to help humanity. On earth there are many different types of jobs in which you can assist others.

You all have a special calling within you!

You decided that to achieve your destiny, each incarnation would provide experiences that would develop a desire for certain knowledge and skills, and you would use these to serve in Heaven. All of you need to listen to the voice in your head, which you can interpret as your intuition, your feelings, and your emotions, and be in touch with your own personal guardian angels. Many angels surround you at all times, guiding you and helping if you ask, for they love you. They are serving you with love and faith.

Be aware that there can be a negative voice speaking to you! We call this the ego. To the unaware soul, ego is known as pride in the way you see yourself in a negative or positive way. When your spiritual vibration gains strength, your ego can react as a spoilt child giving you negative thoughts, which then causes you to react poorly to your fellow human beings, and so guides you away from the Light. If you find yourself cursing, putting down people, and doing the wrong things, and you understand that this is so, you can be sure this is the ego trying to regain the power that it has had over you since your first life began, thousands of years ago. This is one of the most difficult parts of your ascension program. If you are deemed ready by the angels who have watched you develop, then your ego will definitely become stronger and more determined not to let you vibrate in the Light. It wants to be your master! It will fight to be in control! You will need to decide what you are going to do. As always, it is your choice.

The angels will help you when you ask; they will not impose themselves on you. We stress that YOU decide which way this life of yours will go; towards the Light as the I Am Spirit, or stay on earth bound with the ego and its domination of the baser instincts with in you. This will continue until you master your negative ego and choose the Light. We are sure that you will choose the Light that is being shown to you.

You are an advanced soul. Help by choosing and using positive words, actions and love.

Trust, faith, charity, but the greatest of all these is Love.

Blessings to you,
Maitreya

JESUS

I am going to explain why you are moving forward in your journey, for there is a something special in your life that you are seeking. In the past there was not the access to information that there is now, and so if one person saw a glimpse of the Light, they were placed on a pedestal to be worshipped, or persecuted for being different. Now as we say, the information from one point in the world can travel to many other places in a very short time via television, radios, the internet, and newspapers. People now have access to what is happening everywhere. Add to this the education that is available, and the psychic experiences by those who are advancing and have gained aknowledge of these events, and perhaps a special ability. There are many whose vibrations are not high enough and will not accept this is a way of life, and they will claim that those who do are very different. Even though my life was an example to the world and Christians accept this story, they can often fail to see the relationship between my ascension and that which happens to them.

My words, beloved people of mine, are that you are on a journey as I was.

This is a journey to the Light, a journey Home since you are a beloved Child of God, and therefore you are all brothers and sisters of one big family. Love for your fellow man is as important to the mission as you are. You will find that if you love yourself as Child of God, you will love all the people you interact with. Do not judge them! They are on their own journey. You do not know what choices they made before this incarnation. They may have gone off their Path, since they will not have a memory of what life they decided on before birth. They may have a feeling that there is more for them, and they may be getting closer to being aware of what life is about. They could be very early in their lives and incarnations, and still gaining experiences which they will incorporate into their future lives. Just love them as a person due the respect that comes from equality. Ask your heavenly Spirits to guide them.

You will find that a wonderful world is coming.

For those of you on your last incarnation, or nearing it, and those still based in earthly vibrations, a New World is at your door. A prophesied wonderful world filled with love and joy and the desire to help each other.

This New World is not being born easily as change normally moves slowly, but this one is coming quickly causing great contrasts in some lives. In the very recent past, the pendulum went too far into the negative and illustrated the self serving ways of those who were looked to as leaders, and it is now coming back to where it is showing a more positive outlook.

I thank you for the chance to write these words.

Jesus

CONFUCIOUS 14/7/11

This part of the written sermons provided for you will be about the cause of problems for the people of the world.

These personal problems do occur constantly and repeatedly throughout the lives that all are living. We feel that if this is addressed, it will help those who desire help. These souls may feel that they are doing the right thing and cannot see why they do not feel firmly set on their Path back to their heavenly Home.

We will begin with the story of Jesus. He helped where ever he could, but the story of his life, as presented in the Bible, was that he was unfairly treated. This has not taken into account the part of life that begins before birth for every-one. This is a time when you, your guardian angels, and a group of special angels discuss the needs of your next life time. Many of the so called good people do not always have an easy time of life, and this is due to their time of pre-birth decisions that they made in which they intended to increase their knowledge of life.

They are actually on a Path of learning that they felt they needed to advance. Remember that karma is also a part of this plan. Bad karma which has been earned in past lives needs to be rectified throughout following lives, and this time may their chosen time of repaying. The plan that you formulate is the basic one that you will follow. You can journey several different ways, but you will get there.

You have free will to achieve your aim when living on earth, and before birth, when planning this next life.

This planning is done with great joy and anticipation. You are guided by your angels to whatever you have decided to learn, and this is always kept within your capacity to cope. Just follow your plan, step by step, for it is implanted in your soul.

It is commonly said that, "The longest journey begins with a single step", so meet your role with graciousness.

Confucious

I Am JESUS 15/7/11

My dear people, I wish to comment on your life as it is now.

There is a great turmoil in this world with disasters, poverty, violence and war. This is sad, but it was prophesied many years ago by those who were open to their ability to see the future. You have been told that it is a cleaning process for the world, and it is! Do not worry about this happening, as all the people who are involved agreed to be a part of this process. They may not remember their pre-life decisions when they decided that their role was to participate in this part of the world's history. Yes, they are distraught at losing their way of life, but they will recover and go on to a better life, even if not in this one. They are blessed by their Father in Heaven for volunteering for this role. All of you have a part to play, and these roles are appearing as we speak. Do not despair that the world is full of violence, for this will diminish over the years. Those who are involved in this role of darkness have a long journey ahead, as have the new souls on the beginning of their journey, and as you had many hundreds of life times ago. At this moment a great many souls are nearing the end of their journey, and so they are being replaced in a self perpetuating process. The world will continue on, to grow and develop, and so many new souls will come in to compensate for those who are ascending. These new souls will develop and they will be a part of the great New Age that has been described by the angels dictating this book. They too will rise in vibrations after many lives, as you have. Slowly and surely the world will be the wondrous place that we have described.

Stay positive and keep your vibrations up. Even in this troubled environment you can have the wonderful experiences as one of those who know the Secret of Life. Do not read of the evil side of life for this will bring up negative feelings which are self perpetuating. Read of joyful events and stay within your positive social and family groups. This does not mean to ignore others who have not found the way! You will intuitively know of those you can help compared to those who have a basic vibration level.

Be assured that we are with you. You are a loved Child of God, and your Father cares for you, and tends to you and your needs.

"Ask and it shall be given," is a phrase that you should remember.

It is your world now, so do your part and you will grow in spiritual knowledge and stature.

It is your choice my friends.

Jesus

SEREPIS BEY 16/7/11

We would like to tell of many things that are relevant for the novice on their Path.

Things such as the role of karma, vibrations, of angels and their duties, and the role that these play together as you advance in your life. This may be your last life, or one of the last, and all on earth will travel this Path. Eventually karma, both positive and negative, will be an area that will be understood as a payback for deeds that you have done during your lives. This is so, but it is more than that. The lives you live are filled with both negative and positive situations, and the balance is always changing. Karma is deeper than just balancing the situations of the past, for Now is what life is all about. Each person has a Now with a myriad of situations that are to be experienced as they progress during life. When you pass into your final life on earth, please know that you will not be perfect, but your karma will be towards the positive side of the pendulum, and as minimally negative as possible. It is expected that there will be residual negative karma at this stage, but it will be less than in previous lives. With a percentage of your inherent karma left when you become aware, you can consciously remove some more negativity as you intuitively do the right thing. Past dislikes, hatreds, intentional harm, and doing the wrong things intentionally, are a part of your remaining karma that can be worked through with your angels, but you must ask them to help. You may be guided to books, journals, lectures and other areas from which you may gain the knowledge that will help you to forgive yourself for your transgressions.

Heaven does not judge you. You will do this!

Your inner Spirit knows when you have done the wrong thing and so you must be the one to forgive yourself, and love yourself, if you wish to reduce your karma. As you age, you can look back on your life and see the areas that are causing you to hold yourself back from accepting of the purity of your Spirit. Meditation can help you as it opens your mind to higher vibrations and positive thoughts, which then allows this positive action to cleanse your way of life. Once you have an awareness of your Spirit, you then have the ability to naturally behave and live as you should. This leads to an enjoyable life of acceptance of all in your life without stress, and this leads to the ability to function at a higher level. This level is necessary for travelling on your Path for the last stage of your journey.

Now is a wonderful time for you. Not as in the terms of this era of this life, but Now, being the moment that you are living. If each moment is as pure in thoughts and motive as it should be, you will truly experience the spiritual Now that is promised to you.

Take this experience with both hands and be happy, for life is for enjoying. You can show others by example, what it is that carries you on in such a carefree manner. We are always with you.

I am yours,
Serapis Bey

GOD 18/7/11

My child, you will know my name soon. I am known well and will indicate my name to you soon.

I will begin with a saying that is known as, "There is more to Heaven and earth than is known or realized." I wish to add to this saying. You know small pieces about Heaven, but there is more, oh, so much more to this than you can imagine. Yes, it is a truly wondrous place, but do not think it is for indolent people who are self indulgent to their own needs. One does not live through all your earth lives to learn what characteristics are necessary for a fulfilled life, to waste and forget it once in Heaven. Once you have gained your heavenly status, your life really begins.

Life on earth is a preparation for your heavenly work, and here in Heaven you will continue to grow and exceed your dreams and wishes.

A Spirit that arrives in Heaven will be met by loved family members and friends. You will remember your angel assistants from between lives and you will have time to enjoy those from your last incarnation. This can continue until you feel the need to do some constructive work and service for your Father in Heaven. As on earth, there are many occupations that will interest you and which can help people on earth. Our desire is to have as many souls as are able to, to learn their lessons and come back Home.

Then, there will be other new souls who will take their place and the cycle will continue.

The stress that is in your life comes from feeling that you are alone, and that alone, you have to attain certain levels of education, to get the best job available, and receive the highest monetary reward for you to live your life completely. This is not a pleasant way to live and we want you to realize this it is not necessary. You planned the way your life would be! If you can relax and just enjoy Now, and not worry about the future, then you would be will be closer to the heavenly way of living. Along with your work, you will also have time to enjoy the many activities you enjoyed on earth such as the arts, crafts, sports, and outdoor activities.

I cannot fully illustrate what a wonderful time your Now will be when you have finished learning all your lessons of life on earth. There are no words to describe this time, but it is possible that you may have flashes of intuitive memories from your journeys Home in between your past lives.

So I encourage you to be the best person you can by helping others, loving all by learning that they are equal, and by being happy to raise your vibrations ready for your life in Heaven. Not for a quick visit as before, but a new life beyond comprehension at this stage.

My many friends, this will be yours.
(Maitreya told me that this writing came from God).

WHITE BUFFALO CALF WOMAN 19/7/11

I am going to say that all is right with the world to come, but we know that all cannot be perfect.

Only in Heaven is perfection achievable, but I know that you have heard of the fallen angels. It is a pity that evil and wrong doings are every-where but it does not need to rule our world. It is something that can be fought once it is realized. Evil is a fallen Spirit that the ego supports. The ego likes drama caused by fighting, bad deeds, poor behaviour and egotistical attitudes that offend others. The ego is within you all the time, and is not a problem when dealing with the physical needs of the body, such as cleanliness, tidiness, and orderly timetables, but it does not support the Now of life when your Spirit is emerging. The ego wants more and an unseeing person is a puppet for it. You will know that a person is subject to their ego when you feel negative vibrations emanating from them. Ego is the basis of the word egotistical,which means to be dominant regardless of the situation it is in. Egotism is often referred to and understood as being aggressively dominant, but some souls do not have such a nature. Shy people are also ruled by their ego, which causes them to feel that they are not good enough in any way and that they can't do anything right. They then feel inferior to the other people who may be dominant or not. The sick are also ruled by their ego as their negativity perpetuates the disease, the sickness they have. A feeling of hopelessness is what the ego promotes making it difficult to become well. Fear is also the work of the ego. Not the fear that protects you from danger, but fear of competing in life, and of working and enjoying others company. So you can see that the ego can have a strong hold on the feelings of the individual and will use it to its own advantage. The ego within you has been with you all of your life times. It was useful in your beginning lives, for it was a guide to organizing the daily aspects of life so that you could get through the day. As you grow in ability and are finding your inner Spirit, ego does not want to be relegated to a back seat and so it has found a confronting way of controlling all you do in life.

The way to defeat the ego is by ignoring it!

It will still be there trying to dominate your moods and attitudes, but just be aware of this negativity in your life and passively ignore it. Listen to your positive quiet voice within! Think of Nehru Gandhi and his passive protest with his people. He led a passive resistance with his people and the protest worked. You can take this method for your own when trying to diminish the power of the ego over you. Acceptance is what is necessary; not of what it is trying to make you do, but as a passive acknowledgement that your ego is trying to control you. Turn the other cheek and do what makes you feel the positive life force for yourself. Life enjoys the humble person, but not so the shy one, since they cannot be approached, and not the arrogant and dominating one, as they are feared, but the one who enjoys and loves life and all those who complement their existence. Joyfulness in life is a positive force for growth. Caring for yourself and others is a positive force, and with this comes the quieting of the ego's power. This is the way of life that is most rewarding for you. Aim for it and you can achieve it, and the abundance of life will be yours.

Believe in yourself,
White Buffalo Calf Woman

ST. GERMAIN 20/7/11

Here we are together to discuss the ways of being saintly.

It is thought by many that this is the way to gain Heaven's support. It is not really, but that is what has been thought and taught for many lifetimes. What needs to be talked about is humility, and this is to be humble without self degradation. This is really what needs to be aimed for and attained.

When the word humble is used, it brings up the image for many of a shy, reticent individual, with little vitality of life. Also, as some-one who negatively uses thoughts and actions to control themselves, and tries to appear selfless in the eyes of all, even if this is not so! This is a self initiated act which is played by the ego for onlookers. The ego is within and is in charge. To find the real you who will succeed with the heavenly ideals, you will need to live a true life to travel Home. White Buffalo Calf Woman said that the ego needs to be tamed by non assertive means, and this is by using a passive knowledge of it and what it is doing, and how it is reacting in different situations. When this occurs, the ego is dampened down and becomes powerless to rule you and your way of life.

This will open up an awareness of your Inner Being.
Your Spirit is waiting to be heard.

This is your inner self, your Spirit who is your intuitive messenger, sending you the ways of correct behaviour and attitudes so that you can react properly. By properly, please know that there is no absolute definable way that is correct for your Path forward.

Each one has their own way, and your map is imprinted internally and has been there since you were born for the first time. When you find a way that suits you, feels comfortable and you feel that it is right, it probably will be. Travel on this road and be aware of changes that are directed to you, for your inner guidance system will be at work. Be sure that it is not your ego raising its head to lead you astray, but that any change comes deep within the calm centre of you. This centre knows of your plans and is helping you. This is the Spirit within you, and you will know it when it speaks to you in its soft calm voice of reason. Be guided by it and you will become a truly humble person who knows what is right and what is wrong! A truly spiritual person is at peace with them self, their family, friends, and work partners. They are looked up to as a lesson in how to be happy, and one who has had that happiness spread and is seen as a positive vibration of love. The love of living is what your Father in Heaven wishes you to achieve. When this happens you will know it, and feel it, and be grateful for it. Be aware that your angels are helping you as a truly humble person will not assume it is all their own doing, and will know that asking for help is also an acceptable part of being humble.

So you see, by being humble, you will not allow life to walk over you, but you will be a part of spreading these positive vibrations for all who are ready to see and learn from your example. You will be teachers of faith and love in your area of life, and you will receive blessings from above and continue to progress along your individual Path back Home.

I Am,
St. Germain

QUAN YIN 9/8/11

I will begin this first discourse by saying that we are happy with the way that the people of the developed world are turning towards the Light, and away from the past trend of worshipping the materialistic life.

This world of Now is the beginning of the New Age, and you are all part of it. The reason many of you returned to earth at this time was to share your talents with others, and to help and guide the seekers of wisdom during their life. This is your chosen Path, and although it may appear as a difficult time, it is a time as never before. It will be a time of resolution, of intuitiveness, and of a changing mentality towards a positive way of life.

You will find a way that is totally yours and as unique as you are.

You are an individual. Others may be similar but they are not you, so use this difference to help where ever and whenever you can. Where once there was a secret around truly spiritual experiences, now it is quite open and available for all to discuss, to take classes and work for a living in this area. Do not feel that you need to seek to learn in a professional way and gain certificates to enable you to do your lifetime promise. The knowledge is innate, but there are plenty of articles that you can access that have been written, books available, and groups with the knowledge of the Secret of Life, so that you can refresh that which is within you, when you wish.

It is said that together we are a support for each other's flourishing growth, and for love with its positive vibrations that show through in all you are doing. Relax and enjoy your experiences, for once this happens, the door for your angels to answer you will open, and you will find their guidance invaluable. Your growth will happen easily, and any information that you ask for will be sent to you to discover, and this in turn will promote your growth. I will say that not all of you will succeed at your choice of experiences, but each life you lead brings you closer to your final life in which you will be a highly developed soul ready for your next stage. In your final life of innumerable past lives, is the accomplishment of what you endured or enjoyed from the experiences and lessons that you set yourself to learn. With so many advanced souls on earth together, you can see how powerful a tool this is for helping the world's need to have a clean out to ready itself for this initial stage of the New Age. Then will come the Age of the awakening of many Spirits who will realize that they are a true spark of God their Father.

I will leave you with this statement that is directed personally to each of you. You are a truly splendid being who is blessed for all you are doing for this world. We thank you for your dedication, but remember to have fun, for this is not meant to be a dour experience, but a thrilling part of a wonderful life. Enjoy, for this is your time to blossom.

I remain your friend,
Quan Yin

MERLIN 18/8/11

In the future there are to be many times of darkness and Light, for these are contrasts and will always exist.

They exist to show how good is always superior to evil, and this is visible to all seeking the right way of life. You can ensure that you are in the Light of goodness throughout your development! It is your choice, for if your nature wishes to follow love, kindness, and happiness, this then can be achieved by having a positive self concept. There is a great difference between a positive self love, and the egotistical negativity of domination which is shown by an aggressive nature. You are here to choose your way and the Light will guide you. Follow the Light and let it show you the Path to take. If you step off the Path, you will know, for your intuition will indicate this by the insecurity you will feel. Take a step back and re-assess your road and your intentions. Find where you stepped off the Path and return there, for this is where you can stop your small problem before it becomes a larger one that leads you towards the dark.

We angels are with you, and always will be regardless of your missteps.

Be aware to ask for help and intuit the guidance that we send. You are never alone even if you reject us, for we know that you cannot see us in a life that is in the dark. A call of, "Help me!"

always comes in distress, and this will be our signal that you are ready to be helped back to the Light. We will always help you! Take slow steps in the dark, and then as the Light appears, take quicker steps in anticipation of coming back into it. You will never be left to wander in the dark forever, for after such a life, you will have your plan reset and we will show you how to find the right direction.

With love, help and your insight, you will grow with a positivity that is visible to all.

Be as one.
Blessings,
Merlin

SEREPIS Bey 7/9/11

I am here to tell you of the time of mourning, for this is a difficult time to cope for those involved with a personal loss.

The loss of a loved one is understandably filled with emotion and a feeling of devastation. This is an aspect of grief and it is necessary to let these feelings out, for if they stay within, they are self destructive, and so those who keep their grief at a high level are not able to lead their own life. As we all know, happiness is necessary for the growth of the soul, and this is what each life that we live is about. In happiness, we love and rejoice, and we can follow the Path to the right way of life.

You rightly ask us of how you can be happy now that you've lost a child, a partner, a parent or a friend. The response is that a time of grief must pass to lighten your load. To achieve this, you need to be active in your mind and body so that grief's lessons can be learnt. This does not mean forgetting your loved one, but placing them in your mind and heart so they are always there while you continue with life. Life is about independence, of free will and about love for all around you. If you follow these ideals you will flourish like a beautiful rose.

As a rose is made by God, so are you.
A rose is a thing of beauty and joy,
and this too is your role in life.
You are like a rose;

from a bud to a perfect rose,
and with age still beautiful,
but mourned on its death.

Mirror your life on a rose, for it is showing you the way.

You will remember a special rose in your life and be sad at its passing, but it will live forever in its glory in your heart and memory. With the passing of a loved one, think back on their life which was intertwined with yours. You grew together, and in the passing of your dear one, you need to retain their memory as a beautiful event in your life which helped you grow and develop. Be aware though, that this is not the end of their life and it should not be the end of yours. You may even feel your loved one's presence and see little things that present them self to you. Be assured that these messages are sent with love for you. If you believe that they have not died but have just passed to a higher life and level of vibrations, then you can still enjoy these loved ones in your life. Ask your angels for help to communicate with them but do not dwell on this aspect, as it can hold your development back. Just let it be a part of your spiritual development.

The lesson for you today is that you never lose your loved ones. They are with you, a part of you, and inspire the love in you that you can continue to grow on.

Believe, for I am,
Serepis Bey

OSIS 11/10/11

We will start the day with the Meaning of Life for all, for this is what you are all seeking. The Meaning of Life has been debated, but it has not been resolved to the satisfaction of all.

Each of you now realizes that an individual's differing stages of development are responsible for the levels of satisfaction in their life, and so of course, this is where the different opinions form. Then how can it be possible then to help all see that they have a role in their life? This is a role which they pre-set before their birth and with their angels input.

The answer is that the Meaning of Life must be adjusted to the level of development of each individual. A difficult task you say, but think about the very basic ideas that form a way of life that is useful, advantageous to all and filled with kindness. Most people can relate to this perspective, but those who are locked up with, and controlled by the ego, will encompass just some of these ideal behaviours, just as long as it does not affect their life style. Since the ego likes to be noticed, then you can use this to draw these souls closer to their ideal behavior by praising any positive behavior, as you do when training a child.

You see my friend, you can reach most people who have a problem, but know that when a person is living in the darkness, it can very difficult to help and they may need trained professional help. Praising the person, which includes the ego, for any positive behavior, is all you can do, for this is your love being shown. With other developmental levels we can see some of the aspects that give life it's meaning, for without meaning, life is adrift and being wasted. Since you are aware of the Meaning of Life, you shine as a beacon with your light glowing outwards, and this is not missed by any one.

It is a great positive energy that is perceived by others as a bright personality, as a kind nature, and of being a really nice person. You then can draw forth this same positivity from a life that is being led by another. You are teaching by example, and this is so much better than just telling and describing what is necessary. The Meaning of Life is based on love, which is the pure simple love for all of God's creations. This love is not just for people but is to be directed to all He has given to make the world unique, and these creations are yours to use freely. Love comes in many forms such as the love of a parent to their child, the child for its pets, the man and woman relationship, the gardener for their plants and so on, for in every aspect there is love. Once you find this love, you will blossom as a beautiful rose does. You will feel love, emulate it, and give it, regardless of any situation. Love will guide you every moment that you are living. Love is all, and this is the Meaning of Life! To find this love, and to grow and enable others to appreciate and find love is the most important role that you can have. With this love comes the ability to grow spiritually. To realize that God is love, and that you are God's child, is the greatest accomplishment you will achieve in your life. You are now on the Path Home.

This then is the Meaning of Life; to find God's love is within you and to shine it outward.

To know that you are on your Path Home to God, and that you will continue to develop in your spirituality with this as your life's base. You will then be able to sense God and help others in any way that you find you are able to. This is what all are seeking and they will find this state of body and mind as a living Heaven on earth. The Lord's Prayer says, "Thy will be done on earth, as it is in Heaven".

The Meaning of Life then is clear. Follow your Path and if you misstep, you take a step back and then restart. The Path is yours to follow.

For I am,
Osis

ORCHUN 13/10/11

I wish to talk regarding what is and is not. A puzzling statement is it not? No, not when you look at the idea behind this bland statement of nothingness. To begin, we shall look at what is in this world of yours. Look around and you will see so many things that you cannot possibly note each one. So within your life there is a wealth of variety to enjoy. This is good!

Now we need to look at what is not. You ask me, how do I know what is not, when I know not what you are referring to? We are referring to all the things that you want but do not have. These are the things that you have tried to gather to yourself but have not happened. Why is this so? Shall we look at the ways we fail? We fail because the circumstances are not right, or the timing is wrong, or we can't decide what it is we want specifically. When you say that you want wealth to buy all that you can, then you are not being decisive. This is not a precise statement!

All things can come to you if you know how. You are obviously a soul well into your positive identity, for you are reading this book. So you have heard of manifestation but do not know how to use this precious tool? No, it's not wrong to want all the good things in life, for by gaining them you are giving back through financial payments to those who provide them for you. Yes, you need to look forward to your own pleasure, but you also need to replenish the world. You have heard of the statement that says, "What goes around comes around." This does not only refer to karma based behaviours but also to your finances. Money does make the world go round, for when you buy, you will spend money which in turn pays others, who in turn buy, and then pay. The cycle continues, for this is called the economic climate of pay and be paid. Giving is one of the first things you need to learn, and that giving should be done with love. With receiving, there comes an appreciation of the object and a love of the same.

Love is giving and receiving, and we all know that love makes the world go round.

Your needs and wants are the basis for manifestation, but you need to be very specific about that which you want. When you are asking the angels and God for all that makes you happy, do not generalize, but say specifically what it is you want. Writing the request and using a picture can refine your request, but do not tell your manifesting angels of how or when to give you what you want. Heaven works in mysterious ways, so just wait as your specific request is sent to you. You can ask for a reasonable time limit, but remember, do not demand of your angels. Demanding is not the way of gaining pleasure, for anticipation is more than half the joy of receiving. While waiting for your manifestation, you must believe that what you want is actually on its way.

Trust in the process, for trust is a vital step.

It is a vital step, for if you don't believe, how can it come true? Believing increases your anticipation, then anticipation increases your belief and in turn the joy you feel in receiving. It's a very simple formula to remember and use. As long as you stay with this formula, you will find that all is possible! There are so many areas that you are not aware of, but do remember to thank Heaven and give back to the community, or you will find that your source will cease.

It is now yours to use, for this method has been proven many times before. Do not feel guilty about wanting, for this too is what God wants for you. He is your Father, and He wants you to enjoy all He has made in the world. For with joy comes love and happiness, and when this occurs, your vibrations rise and you become more aware of what is around you.

For I am,
Orchun

MAITREYA 17/10/11

I come to talk about the things that concern most people when they are finding their Path. These things are taken very seriously and so we will respond in like manner. We will begin with the aspects of the Path. Where is it? How do I find it, and how do I know when I have found it? The only thing that is known is that the Path takes you to your Father in Heaven.

The Path is a way of living.
It is a way of faith, of trust, and love, and for all this, a feeling of awareness of all in God's world.

You see, it is up to you to find a righteous way of living in which you appreciate all which God has placed in your world. To go Home to God, you need to obey His Laws, all of which are based on love for your fellow man. Respect, love, caring and helping are the pre requisites for this life. Ask and you shall be shown the way, for you are not alone. You can find what you think is your way, but if you don't feel totally comfortable then it probably isn't, and this is when you request help from your angels. That is why you have them with you all of your lives.

Sadly, in the beginning of your awareness they are not often called upon, but they are there to help you begin make sense of what is being shown to you by your own spiritual spark. You have these wonderful angels who are waiting to be asked to help you. It is their greatest pleasure when this happens, and they are with you always as you travel on. As you travel, your awareness deepens until you feel at one with God's earth. Your vibration will increase and then your life really takes form.

With this feeling, you will know when you are on your Path, for you are in tune with the Universe and all its joys. It is a great feeling of awe that is centered in love, for love is what your journey is about.

Today we find that there are many pleasure dominated people who feel that to follow a spiritual Path is to stop doing what they enjoy. This is not so, for on your journey Home, God wants you to enjoy every aspect of life that He made for you. He made life and so why would He not want you to enjoy it? Have fun and do all you want to explore the world and its boundless treasures. By doing this, you will expand your consciousness and see even more than the others who do not appreciate where all this wealth came from. Enjoy yourself, for as long as you are not harming any others, you are living by His Laws.

I am here to tell you of the wondrous life you can have when you find this Path of yours. Everyone has a Path but not all are the same, for God created you as an individual to live life the way you wanted. You chose your life and lessons in between your earthly deaths and being reborn, and you will again become aware of what your role is in serving God and mankind. Your hobbies, interests and abilities are all an indication of where you are going, and every Path is different in this way. The destination, which is God's Home, remains the same for all but it is your ability and chosen life interests that are different. Again, your angels help you decide where you want your interests to take you. All of you will find your way Home and all will serve the world in their own way. God is waiting for you regardless of the amount of time that you take to achieve it. He is patient, He believes in you, He loves you, and He waits with great joy to see you finding your way.

You are blessed.
I am,
Maitreya

SEREPIS BEY 18/10/11

I am going to talk on the subject of what is important in your life. We will begin with the idea that all you do is important! It must be, for you are a child of God, and by implication He has made you important. Yes, we realize that none of you are perfect, for this is a status that is to be aimed for as you grow and advance, and once your Path to Heaven has been achieved you will still continue to seek it. Perfection on earth is a fleeting idea but one must try for it. By aiming for it, you can lift your vibrations and your knowledge of right and wrong thus gaining a balance which is tipped in towards right, which of course is what is desired. Once in heaven you will still be seeking to attain perfection through continued lessons, for this is what your journey is about.

So, we see that your life is important, for once you tip the scales in favour of right behaviour towards your fellowman, then your awareness grows and you get much closer to your final life on earth. This life, the final life is when you are assessed by your heavenly angels, and when the good within you weighs more than the bad, you will be deemed advanced enough to pass to your Home to be with your Father in Heaven. When this happens, He will be so pleased and proud of all you have achieved. He is proud of you and He loves you regardless of what you are involved in, but He feels intense sorrow if you are not achieving that which you promised to do when preparing for this life.

Therefore, all you do is important in your life! Each life is a learning exercise and this is the reason you are incarnate on God's earth. Your life is important, so please believe it. When you were made as a child of God it was decided what your role on God's earth would be, and how this would assist Heaven once you attained this certain level of development. It is up to you to refine your behaviour as you become more in touch with your Spirit that God gave you at the birth of your first life. God gave you the ability to love. As you grow in goodness towards others, you will find love is a great part of your life.

Love is what you are here to learn.

This is the love of a parent for a child, for your partner, for your family, your neighbours, the world's people, and most importantly for God, for He is your Father, your primary Father. This is the most important aspect that you must come to learn, for without the love of God you cannot have love for others on earth. Your aim is to fill your life and all that you do with love.

It is good to love all the population for they are all the children of God, and that is where your equality is.

Don't forget that world holds so much more than just people. Look around, for His wonder abounds. Open your eyes and start to enjoy all that is available to you. Enjoying your life is what God expects you to do. There is a great misconception that to be spiritually aware, one must be a so called "goody two shoes", to quote a phrase often used. This is very wrong, for with this restrictive life style you are not a partaking of this world that was made for you to use. The whole world was made with great love so that you may participate in all there is, so do it. You will be seen as spiritually advanced and you will show to all that you are enjoying all that is given with God's love.

We come to the end of this tale of the importance of your life. We feel we have shown that enjoyment from participation in all of the world activities will lift you higher, and God's love will shine through you and it will reach all the people you meet.

Try it, for you have nothing to lose except an existence in which you are not advancing as you should.

God be with you.
Serapis Bey

ST. GERMAIN 2/12/11

I am going to continue the story that my dear friend Serepis Bey began. Let us look at how this is will happen.

We will start with the statement that there is a great divide between many people, and so to get along can be very difficult. Those who are advanced will try their very best to work in the situations they find themselves in, but there are others who are still in the grip of their ego, and as such are not going to show restraint or helping tendencies. What should to be done is what we need to clarify. There are several ways that can be used, but not each way can fully solve what is needed. You, of the advanced nature, will be the one to set up methods that could be used. You will need to try differing ways, and twists and turns, as you work with the problem. If you are not the only person on their Path in this situation, then you will have another to discuss it and plan what to do. This may ease the situation, for a problem shared is a problem diminished in difficulty.

Let us discuss some ways for you to analyze where you are with a problem. Firstly, look at the nature of those who are holding onto their own ways at the risk of causing upsets with their friends and work mates. Is their ego the problem? How can you help one controlled by their ego if they have no idea that this is so?

One needs to come through the back door so to speak, and show these persons how they are acting, for some will find it repugnant when treated similarly with an imitation of their own poor attitude. Once they do complain you can then tell them why you are doing this, and show them that their way is not a way of resolving any problem. If they accede to what you say about them, you should feel a change in their attitude, but if not, then you need to find another method or ploy. If their ego will not stand for you choosing to tell them about the way they act, and then their reaction may be so great that they will feel that they cannot live this way, and will then move on to where they do not feel attacked and are still in control. Since you have done all that you can to help them fit in with solving the problem facing you both and even showing them how they behave, there will be no reason for you to feel badly about them leaving. It is their choice, and this may even be a learning move that teaches them a special lesson in life. If they confront this same problem over and over and have to keep moving away to start again, then surely they may remember what you showed them when trying to help. This could be a turning point for them to understand that their personality is being dominated by their ego.

The best thing, other than one learning about their negative personality and beginning to look for a better way, is that you did not step outside the boundaries which were set back when you realized you had another's ego trying to rule you. You will have done well if you use these methods to solve a relationship problem, even if you don't manage to solve it.

You have stayed true to yourself. Well done!

We will continue with this topic in all different ways as relationships can be a difficult problems. There are always problems in a family, in an extended family, in friendships, work, in various organizations, or with neighbours, and so you will find the depth that we will go to help in such areas. Stay reading, for our purpose is to help you with any problem, big or small that you have.

I am,
St. Germain

MAITREYA 11/12/11

Dear friends, blessings are upon you, for the world is yours and the living is made for you to enjoy.

As you are living in this specific time, yours is a life in which you are destined to fulfill certain tasks. We are going to discuss what needs to happen. It is said that all men are going to be as one at their so called death, and we want you to know that all men are equal at all times for you were all born of God's Spirit. This is why you are equal, but the differences between the others that you perceive are due to the number of lives you have lived and the lessons that you have learned. You are, regardless of your level of development and others, still equal in God's eye and need to be seen to act with this in mind when meeting and interacting with those who you may judge as lesser individuals.

We find it disturbing that many are still judging others, for this is not the way you should be reacting to your family of God. Are you judgmental? Look at yourself and see if this is true. Do you react negatively to unclean persons, or those who act differently, or those from different nationalities? Perhaps you see those who are unable to help themselves and therefore seem not to be advancing in life as you deem it should be so? This is not a helpful situation to judge another of whom you know nothing about. You are sending negative energy to these souls. They too are striving in their life alongside God and their angels, and since energy is a real force, this is delaying what they can achieve and learn. Stop judging and send positive thoughts to these souls, and you will find that a positive energy will grow and tend to the soul of the other person and to you too. You are not helping your own life goal by taking the position of arbiter of what is right and what is not, for another. Do not proceed this way, for whenever you find yourself judging another for even the smallest item, stop and send good wishes and the respect that one of God's children deserve. This way of counteracting negativity will slowly grow to be part of your attitude to others, and you will find yourself growing in compassion and not giving out the negative aspects that you previously were. Just try and you will find the true way of giving love for all around you. These are God's immutable Laws which state that, "You must love one another", and, "Do unto others, as you would have them do unto you".

We know that you feel that some of the judging of life that you do is just a simple thought that registers within your mind, but please realize that any thought has a powerful energy and has a life of its own once it leaves your mind. This then goes to the person you noticed and registers within their life force and then it grows to affect their self concept. So you must now see that you affect everyone and everything with your thoughts, and so instead of negative thoughts, you really need to learn that it is imperative you send out positive thoughts and ideas into the word around you. Your thoughts do not only grow in force around your area of life, but if you think negatively about someone that you have heard from or about, the same result will occur. Be positive and you will go a long way to doing what God expects the advanced soul to achieve.

As this is our introduction to the skills you need to learn to help the world gain positive momentum, stop and think why we are doing this writing, and why you have picked this up to read. It was predestined between this life and your last, when you were measuring what it was you felt you had learned and what areas you need to focus on in this new life of yours.

Everything happens for a reason!

We know that you have heard that before, and this too is something to believe strongly in, for although you have free will to do in life what you wish, your end result will be the same regardless of which road you take to achieve the goal. All of you who live on earth have the same lessons to learn, but the final job that you choose to do to help the word and Heaven began back in your past lives of learning.

All of you, regardless of which level of learning you are, will attain the gift of ascension into Heaven so that you will continue to learn and give back to others of the world.

So be it my friends,
I am,
Maitreya

CONFUCIOUS 13 /12/11

Welcome dear friends to this talk. This is to be taken as an example of how you can find your way during this time on earth.

To begin with, you need to think about the times that you have had so that you have a reference point. Let us think about this now. To go further in your life means that you need to re-organize and revise what you have done until now. You will of course know if you have lived a true life, for this is one thing that all understand. All know if they have done what is possible in trying to live honestly, truthfully, and with respect for their fellow man. This is the way of showing that you have learned so much from your previous lives and this is what you are here for. Learning is the whole part of living so that you can continue to expand your consciousness towards the true Way of Life. This true Way of Life illustrates that you are an advanced soul and your responses to others will show this. You are all on this earth as a spark of God, and it is up to you to enlarge the picture you have of your role.

Look around and you will see many who are not advanced in the learning of life's rules, and others of such fine repute that they are famous in their own right. Now you can find out through your prayers and your own sensitivities about whether you really are truly correct in your thoughts. God's Will is what His Laws are based upon, and they are quite simple, for love is the only requisite. This love comes in many forms such as love for family, friends, and for those not so close in your life, as a respect at all times for them.

Respect is a form of love.

They are God's souls too, and this is why love and respect go hand in hand. If you cannot love or see some good in a person, or feel some kind of compassion for them, then you have not mastered this final stage of your earthly lives. By looking back through your life when you were not as fully aware of what life was about, did you then feel for your fellow man or did you have a superior attitude that put you above them? If so, you need to make amends, for this compassion you feel now may not be a real feeling but just your ego using the time of Now and your righteous attitude from now knowing God's Laws; His basic Laws on which all depends. Your ego can find many ways to divert your journey by giving you false beliefs, and by telling you that you have reached as close to perfection as is physically possible. Be aware that perfection and purity in any life is a dream that does not eventuate. Instead, when you strive to do the right thing by yourself and others, you are aiming towards perfection. As long as you are sincere in your aim and work and reassess yourself constantly, then this is all that can be asked of you at this time.

This is what Jesus life was about; to show you that you have life eternal as he had. He became an example to all who saw the Truth of his life.

You, as one of the advanced souls, are nearing the end of this basic training, and will be able to take this learning and use it as the basis for your next level of development which is caring for your fellow men. Love is the basic area that God asked you learn, to show, and share, and with this final step of learning, you are ready to progress. You journey will continue on and on as you find different areas that interest you, until the next level of education is available to you. Your travels will be of the greatest delight and will go on forever. You are truly blessed to be in this position. Praise the Lord, for He is mighty and with you at all times.

For I am,
Confucious

MERLIN 14/12/11

To start, we will look at what the Truth is that you perceive.

Is it that there is a God? Is this what you see as the great lesson that you have learned? If so, this is good as it is a part of the Truth that you are seeking, and this is to find your way Home to your God. There is more though, for the whole Truth is a group of ideas that you must assimilate and be able to use in your life with the many people that you interact with.

Another area that you need to adopt in your daily life is that all of God's children are equal and must be treated as so. They must be equal, for they are all a spark of God Himself, and even if you cannot find within yourself to be with these immature souls, remember that they are in fact your brothers and sisters. This part of the Truth sometimes takes quite some time for you to come to the realization that you need to care about all the persons in the world, regardless of how they show themselves to be, and this means that even if they are barbaric by your standards, or seem unable to live life as it was meant to be lived. Remember that everyone has a starting point to their lives and these souls may just be at that basic point of their life. Give them your blessings and say it to Heaven, for this will reach them and promote positive energy to use in their daily life. The rule here is to care for their progress, and to show care, you need to look on them with patience and forbearance.

Now we will discuss the matter of a problem that many find difficult to overcome, and that is when to accept that you are not right? Do you continue doing what has worked for you in the past? In this situation you need to listen to your inner voice as it will guide you truly at all times. You know right from wrong at this stage of your development, and when you receive a message, it should feel right, for your intuition is a strong tool with which to assess the situation that you find yourself in. Strive for perfection in your life and all that you do but do not stress if you miss the target. Perfection is the ultimate life aim but perfection on earth is impossible to achieve, and this goal is still followed after your ascension. We find that if you give all that you can to whatever you are doing, then that is taken as a positive result.

Today is the time of growth for all who have arrived on earth to fulfill God's plans, and you have a role to play, for this is your mission in life.

The world needs help, and with all the resources you have at hand, you can use them, for saving the world is the job that you have. Do it as well as you are able to and we will be satisfied with your contribution. We do not want you to stress over what it is you feel you are doing for service to the world, for this negates that which is good. Offer up your positive thoughts of helping the people on this earth, and with the force of all you who are designated to help, they will multiply and strengthen until the New Age is able to stand alone. This job which you are doing is one of the greatest services that you can give for all of mankind. Blessed are you who serve the Lord in this time of need.

So friends, be of good heart and conscience, for you are truly doing a great service in any capacity that you find yourself in. Be confident and listen to your inner-self for your guidance, and give what you can and all will be achieved for your fellow man.

I am,
Merlin

VISHNU 16/12/11

This is good way to talk to your friends, for a book is passed around and all who are interested can read and discuss it.

Today we will discuss the value of life. You know well that it is a very valuable gift that you have, but do you respect it as you should? By respect, we mean that life has such a great value that it should be cared for at all times. We find that even those who say they do respect life can fall by the way by not actually respecting it at all times. Let us begin with what respect for one's own self really means. This is to care deeply about your outside shell that you call your body. Also you need to care for the internal parts of your body of which you sometimes are not aware of, such as your inner being of Spirit and the opposing ego. This area also plays a role in your everyday life.

Let us start with your body and see if you care for it. Since you are the advanced souls of the world, it is most likely that you are able to keep your body clean, well-nourished and presented nicely garbed for the outside world to see. You also would realize that what you visually present to the world is a picture of what you stand for, with your attitude to life appearing through the type of emotion showing on your face as an expression. With these few areas showing in the presentation of yourself to the world, many will accept you as similar to them or move away if they do not like what they see presented. This is called your personality and it is based on the word person, for if you look in the mirror you can see what others see. Take off your blinkers and really assess whether you are giving an accurate picture of yourself, or are you presenting a picture of what you'd like to be. It is known that you cannot like everyone you meet, but you do need to respect them, for love is a form of respect and this is the main and last lesson you need to learn. Do you look presentable in the front that you are giving to onlookers? If there is something aggressive or angry in your look, you will not be able to attract the persons who have so much to share with you.

At this latter stage of your journey Home, you should be able to present the image of warmth, confidence, and be likeable, and this is what you should work on if you show a touch of negativity in your persona. We leave it in your capable hands to assess this part of you and to change, or to ask for help in changing whatever you feel is necessary.

Now we shall look at your internal workings, the part of which you call your mind. What does the word mind mean to you? Is it the capacity to think and learn, the reason you feel you have a good mind? Is it your intelligence that means so much to you, or the ability to out think others? Whatever it is, you need to take into account the Spirit that God gave you on entering your first life. This is the most important part of you as a person, for it is a part of you that is ever-lasting. Your Spirit never dies. It is the eternal part of you.

Your body is different for each life as you come back to learn, but it does not live forever. It is made anew for each life time, and your Spirit lives within as you are learning the lessons that you come back to master. How do you treat your spiritual side? Are you denying it expression? If you allow it, it will guide you and show you how to learn the lessons you need. This Spirit of yours is the greatest gift you will ever get, and it was given freely to you to use or not as a personal choice. Once you find it in all else that is you, you will wonder why you were unable to access it before. There is one problem to know of before you are able to fully trust the messages that you receive, and that is your ego. The ego within you is the side that works in opposition to your Spirit. Your Spirit is innate, and once you find that you can hear or respond to your inner voice, you will know rightness and travel your Path truly. In your earlier lives, the ego had value as it guided you to care for yourself and to deal with life as a very inexperienced person. It can be recognized in a person you see as not advanced such as the bully, the loud dominating person, and the one you feel is not honest within them self. The ego unfortunately does like to take over and is does not give good advice.

Once you find your spiritual inner voice of guidance, your ego will double and even triple its efforts to rule you.

You will need to be aware of the information that you are receiving and judge it from your developed perspective, which should indicate the type of advice being given. So I say to you that the way is not always clear but it can be found within you, for that still, quiet voice is what you need to listen to. It will never lead you astray for your soul can do no wrong, and if you follow your positive internal messages, you are well on your way Home. The other voice, that of the ego will try to gain your attention, but the negative way it will try to get you to act will be shown by its poor behavioural choices. Stay strong until the ego gives in and you will truly be grateful, for your learning will proceed at a better rate and you will become the person that you are destined to be.

Blessings, for I am,
Vishnu

VUTRIMINONTO 18/12/11

Welcome to my first writing. This is a great honour to be included amongst these great angels who are giving advice to you who are so close to your ascension.

To begin, we will make a statement about the life that you live and why you approach it in a different way to others.

The fact is that you are all travelling different ways because you all have a different project to achieve, and this is beside the main learning journey that you are on. Let me explain, for all of you are equal in God's eyes and all will end up at the same place after developing enough to ascend to Heaven, but the different areas are those of your interests which were chosen by you. Throughout all your lives you have developed various areas of interest and skill, while others have developed interests of their own. When you rise to your eternal Home you will use your interests to help those who need it, and there are such diverse areas that need your focus and help. So as you see that you are made equal in Spirit, you can apply yourself to any area that you wish to. With this knowledge you can now develop in any subject or activity you want, for the more you know about this chosen activity, the better it is for you to be able to select where you want to devote your time.

In the future, you will find that there will be choices put in front of you and you can interact as you wish. These choices are from your heavenly angels who are helping and directing you, to see if there are any other types of activities you can become interested in. It is up to you, but there is no reason to stress about what area you need to develop yourself in, for you have a long time to decide. Even in Heaven you may find another area to develop in, for it really does not matter. It is similar to the children who grow up and always know what they want to do for their future, or those who don't know in early life but still find out before they need to get a job. When you find out, regardless of how long it takes, it will be a great pleasure when you begin.

The idea is to learn all you can about being a good person who is ready for ascension and that means to accept all people as your equal, to care for those less fortunate than you, and to love all around you, for God has given you so much to make your life a pleasure. Share all you have with those around you and others will return the favour and share with you. Sharing is a form of respect and therefore love, and this is the one of the greatest lessons that God would have you learn.

Now that you are aware of the reasons for being in touch with reality you will be able to find out where your ability level is. Continue on friends, for this is your way, and your own knowledge will take you further in your skills and learning so that you will feel and know what is right, and what is wrong. Stay strong and stay firm, for you are developing the skills to do what your intuitive instincts tell you.

To you my friends, I give you the knowledge to improve what you want to so you may continue on your Path to Heaven. All will be included in this knowledge if they want to read this article and follow the details of how, why, what and when. That is why at the beginning I mentioned the sharing of a book as the best way to spread this knowledge, for it is a pre-requisite to learning the type of behaviour and attitude for your ascension into the next part of your heavenly adventure.

Blessings are with you,
Vutrimnonto

SEREPIS BEY 20/12/11

Today I will go to the story of how the transformation of mankind is to be managed.

It cannot be done by Heaven alone and so we need help from all of the souls who are ready and on earth for this purpose.

We will begin with the way of managing life, for this is a huge area that needs to be tackled before any job starts, regardless of what it is. Let us look at the parts of this dilemma and so make the process much easier, since small individual parts are the way to do so. Firstly there is the matter of guidance. Who is going to oversee this task? Of course, God and His angels will from their heavenly Home, for they can see all that is happening and such an overview is of great help. On earth there will be many who seek the right to lead this agenda, but those who demand or bargain for this right are obviously still in the grip of their ego. They want this for the glory it will bring them. The souls who seek their guidance and leadership from God Himself, are the ones who will achieve so much. They are a part of groups of similar people and they do not argue about leadership, but are willing to discuss what is provided for them through contact with God and His angelic messengers. They listen to the messages and know to follow them, for they are the advanced souls of this time of the world. They know that they can help, for they are in touch with their angel guardians and others of higher ratings, and they know that to this job well, they must listen and do what is requested. Why you ask, doesn't Heaven just do the required changes by itself?

This brings us back to the free will that all are given to live their life by.

God and Heaven cannot interfere with anything on earth unless they are asked.

This is God's immutable Law!

So you can see that those who would go their own way are not the ones to lead this world in this New Age that has arrived. Once this group does find the key of asking for help and guidance, then they too will serve the great purpose for which they were sent to earth at this time. There are a great many advanced souls on earth just for the reason of listening, being guided, and doing what they are shown as the way to achieve. You are receiving this information so you may include yourself amongst these advanced souls.

Let us go to the planning stage for this is where your guidance comes from. Of course God knows what is needed and wants to pass this information onto you. Are you listening? We are sure that you are. You have the knowledge that you need to agree to what is planned and then the heavenly souls and angels can help. To do this, you need to listen to the inner voice of your Spirit for it will be your guide, and when you are with a group that you are drawn to by sharing the same standards and interests, you will find that all are on the same wave length. All within a group will have very different skills such as highly developed intuitions: as some will be able to hear and talk God and His angels and this will make it easier to receive the messages and to reply to them. This is the chosen job for those who are able to channel these messages from Heaven. Others have the skill of being aware of messages sent through numbers, music, songs and the infinite other ways that messages are sent to show that your angels are always with you. With the myriad of skills that advanced souls have, you will receive all the messages you want regarding the way to help the New Age dawn more easily, and with your prayers, it is a very positive force and much stronger than you realize. When distressed with a problem, all will call out to God for help regardless of their standing in this world. So with the problems that can be seen in this world as shown through the media, many are calling out to God to help. This is their role to play. Your role is the same, but because of your special knowledge, you know the strength of what you are praying for and asking precisely to be fixed.

So you see, that all together you can help God and His messengers to guide this wonderful world of yours to this special Age that has literally started on earth. Altogether, and with the skills of and those in touch with their Spirit and perhaps some psychic abilities, the way is much clearer for all to participate. The only way that this cannot happen is if any ego is let into the scenario, as this is a negative force and it is this earthly negativity is the problem now. Do not let it grow in strength as you have the power to do so much! It was for this reason that you chose to come back in this life to help.

With this guidance, your positive attitude and your prayers, you will be sent blessings, and those of the future New Age will applaud you for what you did to set the world on an even keel. Once this has occurred, the advancement of many more souls will occur and the life on this earth will be as it is in Heaven, and how it was meant to be.

Blessings,
For I am,
Serepis Bey

ORCHUN 22/12/11

I am going to discuss what is necessary for those of you who do not quite understand what it is they are meant to be doing.

This relates to the many people who are having their eyes and heart opened to the idea that there is more to life than they realized. They have always felt that there was more, but only as an internal restless feeling. This is quite normal and is the beginning of an awakening to what really life is all about. Through this life and the others that they have had, they are about learning to be a person who has love within and a respect for all in the world. Let us begin with the reason of why this happens at this stage of their life. These souls who are finding themselves restless, are nearing the completion of their learning and do not feel that life is giving to them all that it could. This is because they are ready to learn the Truth of why they live, and their Spirit is beginning to be felt within as it is growing in strength. This realization occurs for those who are very advanced, and some-times this feeling is with them from an early age. Not many are born remembering this knowledge, but those who do are very blessed, for they can begin their special learning so much earlier and find what it is that they have chosen to do to serve mankind. So we find that there are many degrees of awareness within all the advanced souls, and they are all working on an area that they feel a need to know about.

Let us look at the way that some find out what is known as the great unsung Truth of Life. Since you all have guiding angels, it is easy to understand that they play a big part of when you find that you are here for a purpose. The angels guide you to areas of life that you discussed with them before incarnating in this life, and so when you feel compelled to try an aspect of life that is different for you, you can be sure you are being directed there. In these circumstances, you will be given or shown little pieces of information regarding this life that you are seeking, and when you see it, your interest will grow and lead you down the path of knowledge. When you start finding out about this Truth, you will continue to follow the links that take you further with your interest, and then you will most likely diversify or study in one particular area. This is fine, for you are still learning and extending this particular area or widening your understanding of the breadth of the subjects you are finding. Some of you will discover your inherent skills which are part of the world of God. These skills may include being able to hear those in the heavenly world, or talking to them as our writer does, or of being aware of the future and what it may hold, for the future is not set. As well, there are those who use music and art to lift the vibrations around them, for this is beauty of the highest type. When you start to delve into the so called psychic world, there are a myriad of skills that are available to all, and some, or one of them, will be become highly developed.

It is a wondrous feeling to use these special talents to confirm to yourself that you are not day dreaming but are truly in touch with the higher world of God.

So my friends, this is the time of learning that you can really develop and allow your Spirit to be the great leader it is. It has been waiting a long time to known by you. It has always been one with you, but joyously, you have become aware of it. Your Spirit is the part that has continued through the many lives you have lived since your first one. It is this area that is raising your vibrations to a higher level, and when you are listening to what it tells you, and you learn from it, you are travelling on your Path back to your Home. This is the true Meaning of Life, and it is yours to grab with both hands and live the life that God wanted for you from the beginning. This is His Great Plan; for all in the world to attain their ascension and return to be in their true Home.

Once you find the Meaning of Life, it is up to you, for it is a great responsibility that you take on. You will be helped if you ask God and His angels, and so there should be no stress, but a great feeling of joyousness within your being. This is what it is all about!

You have found the Secret of Life.

Blessings be with, you my friends.
Orchun

MERLIN 23/12/11

Our journey is on its way, for you are learning well.

This book is constructed to show you small exerts from the wide amount of knowledge that is available. The subjects that we your angels have chosen are some of the areas where many of you are finding small or large problems. Many of these exerts are there to support each other, for these different viewpoints, or styles of writing, and expression, are accepted by different people at different stages of their development.

As you read through this book you will find the writings that will help you explore your concerns more fully. This is the stage where you can take your research further or you can decide that you have enough information to deal with this problem by yourself. We wish to tell you of the way of the world, for it from this world that you take your learning. This learning helps you further into developing into the type of person who has modest needs and is happy within them self. It is because of this love they have of self, that they are able to love and respect and give back to others. This is what all on earth are trying to do, for with God prior to birth, they decided what lessons that they should learn and how to deal with the subject of karma.

Karma is a total subject by itself and we will go into this area in only a light way at first. Karma is something that all possess in varying degrees, for what you have done in your last lives will, and does have an effect on how your present life will be lived.

Karma can be good as well as bad, and this point needs to be understood.

Many think that karma is the result of negative behaviour from the past and needs to be repaid to the person to who was slighted back then. Alternatively, you can be positively repaid if you gave of yourself to others in the past! It may have been a small favour that you did or a very large one which caused you a great deal of self sacrifice. In return of such a deed, karma will be in a direct comparison to the goodness you did. There are many people that seem to be lucky, and they will agree but not know why this is so. Some will research their past lives with the help of their angels and try to find why this is so, but unfortunately, others who take luck as their right will gain more karma if they are not careful of how they behave. Karma is relative to the original cause. With the understanding of what karma is and how it works, you should all think twice about what you are doing and how you are towards others. If you are not living as God showed you with the life of His only begotten son, then you can be sure that you will receive back the same type of attitude as you give to others. You must experience all the types of life styles if you are going to be aware of how it is to live properly, respectfully, and with modesty and a love for self and others.

Does karma ever finish you ask? No, not on earth, but as you go further down your Path you will be more aware of yourself as a person of God and you will not incur the strong karma that takes many lives to repay. At your last life on earth, your karma will be totaled up and balanced, and if it is well into the positive side of the scale you will be exempted from paying back much more. If you do transgress badly, then the balance will go back into the negative and you will have to return to another life to amend the problem. At this stage of your journey it is most unlikely to happen, but be aware!

So now that you know about the ramifications of what you do with your life, you need to be aware of how others see you and judge you. It is not necessary to worry about this idea of karma. Accept that this was a part of your other lives which has gone to a greater degree, and know that there is only Now.

So to you I say, let the story begin with and end with you doing the best that you can so that you do not bring any unpleasant karma onto yourself. Since you know that what you do causes karma, then be aware of all that you do, for it is in your hands. Of course you can aim to gain positive karma and this is a wonderful thing to aim for. You will gain by giving love and help to those you live with and those who are part of your life.

I say to you, blessings are with you,
For I am,
Merlin

KRISHNA 25/12/11

Welcome to one of the holiest days of the year, for Jesus was born to show you how to live your life. Use Him as your model and you will not stray from the true Meaning of Life.

We will begin today's writings with the statement that all is well with you and your family, for today is also about your family. Family is love in the deepest way, for it is founded on two souls uniting and creating a new life for a soul to be placed in so that they can then continue their journey, as you are doing. Love is what God wants you to feel deeply in this world, and when you find the right partner and have children or not, you experience the love that enters the core of your body. It is such a sublime feeling for you are actually feeling a part of the heavenly love that abounds for all. This type of love can be duplicated for all to share if you just listen to God's words. He was very explicit when He gave His Commandments to the world. There are ten rules to which you are directed to use as a guide for living your life. Two we are sure you know well are, "Love your neighbour as yourself", and "Do unto others, as you would have them do unto you". These are very straight forward and therefore easy to understand and surely easy to follow. Do you follow these little things, these basic rules?

With the love for your family, you do know what extreme love is, and it is this love that God has for you, His children. You are all His children and so that makes you all brothers and sisters.

For those of you with brothers or sisters, you know that they can be annoying and you can disagree with them, but for most of you, you do love them. This is the same relationship that that God wants you to have with all of those in the world, where disagreements will be seen as verbal problems and not as wars that are imposed upon Nations.

Can you see now that the world's relations should be built on a love; love that recognizes that they are people like you with the same feelings of love for their family and friends?

Respect is another form of love that can exist between Nations even though you do not know them. It may be that you do not understand these people who are causing problems in the world, but you do know that these souls are gaining a negative karma in this life. They can be seen as less advanced souls who are not aware that life that should be lived so that one can grow spiritually.

There are many living who are not Christians and they do not use the Commandments that you have been given to use, but remember that there are many other forms of religions in the world, and if you studied them, you would find that there are many similarities. The main problem is when religiously based people interpret their religion wrongly and use it for their personal supremacy over all those who will follow. This is obviously a less developed soul who is in the grip of the ego, and does not care for any one or thing except the ultimate power of selfish gratification. This is what we are seeing in pockets of the world and it is causing a lot of hatred between the cultures. No, you cannot let the situation stay as it is but you can understand why it is happening, and by sending prayers full of positive vibrations, they can be directed to these areas of misery. So my friends, you can help these poor souls in their troubles, and because you know why this happens, you can still respect them as being your brothers and sisters still living in their early lives. They do need to grow spiritually and many will experience great karma for their next lives, but all have to take the responsibility for the gift of freedom of choice. With this comes a negative karma based result for those who make a wrong choice.

So help your world family with your prayers and respect, not for what they are doing, but for who they are.

Blessings, for I am,
Krishna

MAITREYA 27/12/11

Today I wish to speak on the subject of the Time of Revelation.

This time is coming, and indeed it has already started, as many are aware by observing what is happening in the world.

We shall talk of what is happening, so that if you are unaware, you will then be able to see the signs too and be able to be a part of this message from God. To start with, we will refer to the way of the world now and what it seems to stand for. When you look around, you may see little to encourage you as to the way that the world is going, and you will know that there is a lot of trouble within the confines of many lands. What can you do? This is the question that many caring souls ask. This appears to be a very difficult question to answer, but it need not be, for the way of the world is changing and you are here to be a part of it.

Let us speak of the happiness that is showing throughout areas of the world, for this is part of a new caring for each other and of helping the down trodden who are unable to help themselves at this time. This is what the world is turning to, a world of care and love for each other. This is where the focus should be, for this happiness and a caring respect gives forth positive energy which continues to grow and grow, until those who have been helped then return the favour to others. As the wheel turns, the stone rolls on, and all begin to act as one. Can you see what a glorious future the world has for it? A Heaven on earth is how this joyous time is referred to by the many who are watching the slow growth of love for all in the world.

What about the other side of the world's life? This is causing strain and fear for those who are watching through the various media. While you fear what is happening, and your concern is real and based on wanting safety for the world, your feelings do promote a negative energy which grows just as the positive energy does. The love and fear in the world is so unbalanced, that your task is to swing the pendulum to the positive side and so help the situation that the world finds itself in at this time. To stop the negative energy from growing is quite really quite simple. If what you observe and comment on to your peers takes the form of negativity, it therefore helps the bad situation to grow, so turn your focus away from the media stories of war, fighting, and death, and you will not be assisting a focal point of negativity. Turn off your television, do not read what is reported on this subject in the papers and do not discuss the subject, for if you do this, then no negativity can grow to aid this type of behaviour. Obviously you are aware of what is happening, so send prayers to those who are involved in trying to change the situation.

Prayers from all of you are a very powerful tool!

Think about the miracles that have happened after prayers seeking help have been offered. Look at the church hierarchy who seek proof of miracles from one before they can become a Saint in the church. Miracles do happen and they are directly related to prayers, so follow this way of helping and you will be amazed at how things can turn for the better.

There are some of the population who are directly involved in aiding the cause at its root, but not all are meant for this role. The way that you are being asked to contribute is to pray and provide the energy and permission for the task to be undertaken by the heavenly hosts, for it is their job to support the situation and take it to its positive ending.

So you see my dear friends and helpers, you are here in this time to help in any way that you can, but remember that everyone has a different task to do. All of you need to seek the aid of your angels, for this is what they are waiting for and it must happen before they can do their job. Stay strong, remember to pray, and in particular stay happy and enjoy this life you have, for this is what was meant for you in this life. Send out positive energy wherever you go and you will know find that God is always with you.

Blessings my children,
For I am,
Matreiya

VISHNU 29/12/11

Welcome friends, for today is one for telling the real story of the way in which the past has influenced the future, which is this moment of Now that you live in.

We all know that there is only ever the moment of Now, but we also need to be aware of the past and what lessons it has given to those who understand that today's Now is determined by the past.

Yes my friends, we are talking of history, and though many do not attach much significance to this area, it remains a vital part of today. Free will was the cause of the past days and it is the same for today's history in the making. God gave all of you free will to do what you determined you wanted to, and this trail of self determination is what makes history. For together, many souls can make their wishes unite and this can have the power to move a mountain, as it is said. So you can see, history is a way of finding out what may happen to you in your life and your family's life.

History is very important, for it is a guide to the type of behaviour you should have if all is going to work out well for you in the areas of life that are important to you. We are now going to look at the past to see what actually made the situations that caused a great deal of problems for the world, such as the wars of the last century. These wars were the result of certain ego based attitudes by the antagonists of the time. Many deaths of young men and women could have been avoided if only the proper insight was given to the emerging problem in Europe and elsewhere. Men have a tradition of fighting to dominate another power, and it is such a very deep seated urge that many do not stop or think about the consequences. This is what happened. The youth were called to serve in the army by those who ruled the countries and the armies, and these men did not think further forward to the cost of the end result. Yes, a lot of antagonism came from the other side, but surely with a little restraint, the best thinkers could have got together and master-minded a positive plan to follow. Both sides were at fault as they did not go deeply into possible solutions together with the other country. The result was two dreadful wars and many battles in the last century which killed many innocent souls and caused such misery for these families. It caused poverty for those who were left home to survive and to keep the war effort going by providing the food, and clothes, and the tools of war. The war effort also caused those involved in the bitter fighting to lose faith in the system and themselves. The lessons learned for the world were intense and long lasting, and what happened still lives on in the minds of many.

Later, in the Second World War, the memory of the result of the disastrous atomic bombs that were dropped on Japan has deterred other more recent threats to world safety. There have been other big and small skirmishes in the world but many have been worked upon to solve the problem. We hope that there will be no more world wars for an advanced type of destructive technology is available to nearly all countries, and this should be a great deterrent. History has spoken and we should be listening!

Today, there is still a problem in the world, but the Nations are talking to each other instead of just fighting. This is a control which is being imposed with the great Nations talking to each other, and many alliances are being made, some of which are tentative, and others that are stronger.

The past has influenced this time of Now and this is how it should be for all who live in the world at this time. So I ask that you look about and see if there are any problems that need fixing, and look to the past, for history as may help you solve them. History does not need to be from hundreds of years ago, for history happened as late as earlier in this day, or yesterday, or last week, and so you do not have to search very far to discover a solution.

Learn from your situations, which are given as a way to learn and grow so that you may advance in your life skills. There is help all around you, so look at what is available and use what you can, and your problems will be easier to deal with.

My friends, I am,
Vishnu

ST. GERMAIN 31/12/11

Happy New Year, for you can make it so my friends. This is because the will to do good or evil is within you and you have all been given free will to use your abilities as you wish.

The glory of God is your aim, but when faced with a choice your decision will be unchallenged by God and His angels. Your free choice was given to you at your very first life and is now and always with you, so you can see that regardless of what you do, the onus lays with you. You cannot divert responsibility to others as a child would, but you have total responsibility for all that you do and all that ensues from it.

We will look a little deeper at what has been said, for it is here that many do not take their free will with the responsibility that they should. All that you do in each life is your choice, and as such, gather an impact on the next ensuing life. This of course is called karma and it can be good for you or it may be a problem for you to master in this life. Usually karma is thought of in a less happy way as many think that karma is bad for you. Look at the signs written in shops which say that karma will come to you if you steal from them. This can be seen as a scary event for the sensitive souls who are not of a type to do anything wrong. Those who do steal are usually not put off by the thought of karma as a result of what they do for they do not feel remorse when doing the wrong thing. Karma will eventually come to them, but this karma is not just a bad happening, it is really a teaching aide. As with children, if they are rewarded instantly for the good they do by words or deeds and reprimanded when they err, they are learning right from wrong. Since resultant karma is not immediate to the deed and is often in another life time, many forget what they have done, and when they encounter similar behaviour sent to them, they become upset and complain that it is not fair. There is a warning for that which is not acceptable as it is often said that, "What goes round, comes round." If this statement can be linked to the idea of karma, then all will understand that whatever your free will leads you to do, then the same will return to you and you will experience what it feels like to be helped or wronged. The idea then is to think deeply about what you want to do and decide if it would cause harm or distress to another. It is in your hands whether you will experience negative karma! Positive karma is not thought of as much as negative karma, since people do what they feel is right just because it feels right and good. You also earn this karma in relation to what you do. Those in the world who are devoting their whole life to serving their fellow man will have this need imprinted deeply within them, for this is what they chose before they were born. Past experiences have led them to this life's rewards and they will earn positive karma according to the level of self sacrifice and the level of love with which they do their work. Work is not a term for the life of these souls who are nearing, or at their last life, but it is seen as the journey on their Path that is leading them Home. They chose to do this activity because within them they felt a need to help. This freedom of choice is in action which then leads to positive karma. So you can see that the end result of karma is tied to your own free choice! You need to be aware of what choices you are making and the end results for the others who are involved. If you weigh up what you are doing for the resulting positive karma that you think you will earn, then you are not using free will in the correct way.

To gain positive karma, you need to be doing something spontaneously out of love and the spirit of giving for mankind and its benefit.

The free will you have needs to be tuned into and then you can give with love for your fellow man. You will then continue your journey back to God, your Father. Treasure your free will as a gift from God, and use it wisely until it becomes second nature for you to be kindly and loving to all you interact with. Karma rests with you.

"Do unto others as you would have them do unto you."

Our blessings are yours,
I Am,
St. Germain

MAITREYA 1/1/12

Welcome my friends, to a New Year. I pray that you find it as interesting and as enjoyable at is meant to be for you all.

We will start our talk today by saying that you are all wonderful and are well on your way to your reward. Our talk will be regarding a way of living your life in this fast world while still retaining the ability to be your own self, and not be coerced into feeling that you have to do things that you do not really condone. Business today appears to be ruled by the type of person who appears to have few scruples and will do whatever they need to do to win. They seem to say, "Look at me, I have made a lot of money for this business," but they do not really care about how it was made and at what cost to others involved. We realize that you have to compete in today's business world for it was chosen by you to gain experience of this area, but please understand that you do not have to behave in such a way that it offends your own principles. There are always methods to counteract this type of negativity. It is a negativity, even if it is making money for the business, for it is not a morally right way to achieve!

Let us discuss ways that you can use to forward your business so that it returns a profit, for this is what business is always about. To begin with, you know that you are an advanced soul, for if you weren't, you would not be aware enough of these problems. You would not have such a developed conscience and so would be doing business the same way as those you are in competition with. You may ask me about how a positive conscience can operate with those of a suspect morality? The answer we are pleased to give you is to ask for help, for you know that your angel guardians are with you at all times to help as long as you state where you need the help and the outcome that you would like. You know that you must ask for the things that you want manifested in your life and this is the same thing.

Watch for signs of guidance by listening to your inner self and continue to ask for the right way to be shown to you, and it will happen.

You will find that by having divine guidance in your business life, you will have a business that can be run on faith. What you need to do is being shown to you so that you do not have to function at the lower levels of the mind, as a lot of your competition does.

You do not, my friends, have to sell your soul to keep abreast with the business world, for it will be to you that others will be looking. The others will find that they have gained a poor reputation, while you will be admired for being a truly honest but still an adept business person. It will be to your door that those who wish to do business will come, and also the right type of associates who will enhance what you do.

My friends all this will happen, for you have the faith and trust in your heavenly helpers. They listen to your requests and do what they do well by setting up plans that can only end in good for you. Remember that those managing and working in opposition businesses are likely to be run by those who are still dealing through their ego based mind, but you can be an example to those who are close to stepping onto their Path back Home by just demonstrating the correct alternative ways that are available.

So dear friends, use all the tips on living that you find in these writings to guide you on your life's journey. This is what these writings are for, to make life decisions easier for you, for all that is written in this book is for you and others of your similar development who are awaking to this journey.

Blessings my friends,
I am,
Maitreya

VISHNU 2/1/12

Dear readers, I will tell you about the time before you leave this earthly life for the heavenly area where you will start a new journey.

We know that all of you will come to your last life and so this writing is for those of you who are reading and learning about your mission in your last life. This life may indeed be it; the one that you will progress from. What an exciting idea for so many of you! You have had a long, long time to advance to this stage and so we ask that you enjoy it fully. We are sure you will, but do not worry about what is expected of you for you are going well and we know that you are doing the right things to be at this place and time in your life. Your round of karma will be balanced enough to the positive side, for you have done the right thing and taken any karma and worked with it. This percentage will be positively balanced well above halfway to help you remove any leftover negative attitudes that you may still have. Many of you are above this level, but no one person can be at one hundred percent, for perfection is not gained in this journey on earth. Jesus showed you that, he, as the son of God was as close to perfection as is possible on earth. God has asked you to follow Jesus' way as an example but He does not expect you to be perfect. Your aim needs to be similar to Jesus righteous way of life and this is important to show how well you are learning your lessons.

Over the many lives that you have experienced you have gained a lot of skills, but there have been times that you have also slipped and lost some of what you were unknowingly trying to master. Life has been full of ups and downs and roundabouts, while you try to find what it is for you to learn. These lessons were decided on during your time in Heaven between lives as we have said before. So you are a big part of choosing what it is you need to master. Indeed, this is free will at its most interesting. Many times during your lives you are put with the same people you have had issue with, but in changed circumstances and different relationships. Have you ever felt a feeling of knowing towards a person that you just met, and recognize feelings of love or enmity? This person will most likely be part of your learning from a past life together.

Look how this gives you a head start, for by just listening to your quiet inner voice you can be aware that this person is in your life for a reason.

You will indeed find that there will be many persons from past times, but not all are necessarily there for negative or positive karma. Just know that this is your journey, but that you do not travel it alone for God is always watching you and will help you if you only ask for help. Once you know that God exists and that He is in your life, He will assist you when you call. His angels are always there for you, including your guardian angels who have been with you since your very first life. If you find a choice difficult or you have made a wrong turn, then all you do is ask and they can help you in any situation you find yourself in. There is just one area that they cannot help and this is if there is a direct lesson you have been set to learn. Do not feel that they have deserted you, but understand that this is a lesson which is necessary for you to learn. Take heart, for if you find yourself out of your comfort zone, you will be helped and the lesson kept to be learnt later.

The final lesson is to love all mankind as you love yourself, and once you truly show this to God and His helpers you will find that only minor lessons need to be looked at, and by this stage you will have the ability to do the right thing in many situations. See what a wondrous life you can have as no harm can come to you? You are one of God's children, and as such you are under His protection and always safe. He is waiting for your final journey Home to Him and there will be such rejoicing when you arrive.

Worry not my friends, for now you know what is ahead; infinity is your way and you will always exist.

Blessings to you,
For I am,
Vishnu

KRISHNA 3/1/12

This is the time of the beginning of the age that has been written about and prophesied for many years, or really ages. You are the ones chosen to lead the world forward, and as such, you are being readied now.

How is this is happening? The answer is that you are an advanced soul, as many of your group are, and so have come to earth at this time to fulfill a need. This need is to help the world to begin its journey to a new way of life which will be based upon love for all. If you remember, the last writing told you that the final lesson that you need to learn on this earth as you travel Home, is that of respect for all people, as it is an aspect of love. God sent you to learn about love and all your lessons have pointed to this. You needed to learn how to interact with all the different nationalities and all the different personalities, and you needed to learn to respect and love for yourself also. Without self love, no one can learn to love others, so this is the first love that you need to learn, but remember that this is not the ego driven self love that many people have.

You need to be free of your ego's control so you can gain a self worth that is real.

Real self love does not want to control or tell you to behave in a way that you know isn't correct. This is your ego still trying to have control over you! We know that most of you are past this point in your awakening and so the love you feel for yourself is real and true. This is God's love which was implanted in you all those lives ago when you first started on this amazing journey back Home. This love that is in you, has guided you when you intuitively listened to your quiet inner voice. At this stage of life, you should feel or know that this quiet voice is talking to you. With this guidance and the angels to help you, you will do what is right regardless of the situation that you find yourself in. Since you are so close to your final life on earth, you will find that you have an abundance of love within you and you will find that it bursts out of you with a lovely glow.

This type of person we have described is here to lead the others who are still seeking their way, and there are many more at this time of the world's journey; more than has ever before been on earth at the one time. Your warm loving glow and the way it radiates from you is what shows your way to the future by using your moment of Now. As the time passes, you will find that others will join you, and you will see such a change growing around you with the gathering those who feel drawn to this life of help, respect and love.

This cannot come to pass immediately but we realize that this is the first step. In the past years from the nineteen sixties, the young stepped out of the old traditional way of living and they found what love was about. As any new idea, it went too far, but now the balance is perceived to be right for the next stage. This time of balance or imbalance is how the world moves forward. This is the work that you have been developing yourself for and this is the time for you to do whatever you have chosen to do. All of you have different ways to follow. Some ways may seem to be more in depth than what you are doing, but in the whole picture that God has drawn there will be a beautiful balance with all the different natures involved, and all the different areas that are being helped.

This then is what you are all here for, so my dear friends so, "Go for it", as the young say today, for it an apt expression. Express the love that you feel for God through the deeds that you do. Your journey just needs a bit more of this life you live, and then you can acknowledge that you are accomplishing what you set out to do from that very first life you lived on this earth.

Blessings my friends,
Krishna

MERLIN 4/12/11

It is my wish to speak to you today on how to exist in this world that can be so punishing if one does not respond in a typical way.

What does this mean you ask? Let me tell you about the story that will explain what is truly meant by this statement. To begin with, and there always must be a starting point, we will look at the way in which you interact with the world. Just as everyone does, you say, but why is it that others find that nothing goes wrong, no matter what they do, while you still have the problem of making a right decision. Can we put this down to the karma effect or to the differing levels of development that are inter-mixing? Well yes, all of these are woven into the thread of your life, and are relevant to what you do and how you do it in differing situations. There is though, a wider picture to look at and this needs to include all of the things that you desire and the things that you want to do. To try to look at only one area is not the way to progress with your plans. We will try to show you in a fairly simple way. The way forward needs to be thought about carefully and then the steps planned, for only then will you have an idea of what it is that you really want. If you have wanted something and then changed your mind a few times, this then will cause a problem in conveying exactly what it was you are after.

Yes, it is manifestation that we are talking about, and you need to be very clear on exactly how you want this matter in your life solved. You cannot say that you want to win a lot of money, for this is not specific, and you must leave a certain amount of time for the angels of manifestation to decide how, where, when your request will be given. The only issue for you to decide with utter clarity, is what you actually want and then give a generous time frame for this to be accomplished. We realize that if you want money, and please know that there is no harm in this, you cannot say how this money is to come to you, for the manifestation angels have marvelous and untold ways to deliver this to you. If you have a situation that you want fixed, then you need to be sure where the problem is and what the problem is, before you ask for help. If you have the problem wrong, then the answer that you are seeking would most likely cause more of the same trouble. Once you find your problem and are definite about it, then you can ask for help. Give your angels leeway to fix the cause of the problem. This can cause some more problems but it will only as a required part of the solution, so be patient. Trust and faith are very necessary in the process of manifestation and gaining help.

You all know that you need to ask the angels to help you, and when asked, they will do what they are able to do for you. When it comes to something larger or more difficult, you will need the patience to wait with faith and trust for this to come through. If you have what seems to be a problem with karma, then you will feel that this is for you to attend to also, but ask and you will receive help in perhaps a way that is different to what you may have expected. The end result will be that you will be guided to do what is needed. There is a difference between a karma based need that needs to be attended in this life and a need for other things that you feel will give you the quality of life that you want.

So you need to look at what it is you are seeking; the help for a life lesson, or the fulfillment of a need. This is why you need to be very specific as to what you want, or you may get what you think you wished for and find that it did not solve anything. Money and material goods may make your life miserable for there could be ramifications that you did not foresee. You could be left by your acquaintances who could feel they could not live your life style or, others who become jealous of your new life style. The warning then is not to be flippant as to what you want, since the asking of the angels of manifestation is a serious step in your life. If you do not handle the rewards of your new life well, then the implications are that you may be setting yourself up for more karma and not of the positive kind. By using manifestation as a positive learning experience you will gain positive energy.

When you ask and receive, then the onus is on you to give back to others.

This is the Law of Manifestation!

This must be attended to or you will lose all you have gained. So it comes back to you to be sure of what you want and when you approximately want it, and then spread your luck around. When you receive money, you need to spend, for you are spending money which goes to another who in turn spends, and this is how the economy keeps going. This is how you share your good luck with some who may not know the Way of Manifestation. This is what is meant by the saying, "To spread the wealth".

Now you know the way to move on in the world just the same as others you see. Real wealth can be the cause of, or the result of improperly used benefits. Watch in your own life and if one is ready to know your way of manifestation, then feel free to tell them, for it really is not a secret but is available to all to use. Spread the word but reveal the guidelines too, and all will be well.

I am,
Merlin

ORCHUN 5/1/12

We are going to discuss the way in which some souls can hear us easily and others cannot, no matter how they try.

It does take some time for those who feel they are not able to reach us, but actually we are there all the time for whoever talks, prays, or asks for help. You do not have to hear our words speaking to you for there are many ways in which you can receive our messages. Just to show you that we are with you, we can leave a white feather around as our symbol or you may find five cents on your daily round. These are left as indications that we are always with you, so whenever you see these signs, pick them up and realize that this is your own special connection. Signs can be otherwise shown through the radio or the television, or a sign in a shop. This method of reaching you will be repeated often. You will hear the same song with relevant words until you understand that this is a message. On television, the same thing may happen as a picture or words may continue to appear until you are able to make sense of it. Others have read books and wondered why the same idea continues to appear, and so if you put this to what you have been asking, you just may indeed have your answer. There are a myriad of ways to receive messages that can help you in a predicament, to soothe you, or just let you know that your angels are with you!

These methods depend on you being aware enough to pick up on them, and this in turn will stimulate your intuition which then causes you to pick up the sent messages more quickly as you experience this inner feeling of awareness.

With this awareness comes an opening of a channel within you through which you may start to have such abilities as hearing the heavenly voices, seeing into the possible future, and all the skills that you have heard of but felt shut off from. You do need to know that these are really not talents but are a part of your life and should automatically grow with your development.

These abilities are there, for everyone has them and can develop them to a greater degree.

Not everyone has the same skills, for you are each individuals, and as you vary in your likes and dislikes of different areas, so it is with these skills of communication.

You ask how to develop your skill and how will you know what it is you should be focusing upon? Look back at the types of messages you received when you were just becoming aware, and this may give you an indication of where your talents lie. Meditation is a good way to start opening your mind to any messages or input from your angels, for this stills your busy mind and allows your inner being to talk to you. The voice will be very quiet and almost imperceptible at first, but with continued meditation you will start to hear the voice. If hearing is not to be your way then meditation will still quiet your mind so that you will be able to find different methods of gaining contact with Heaven.

Start reading, for there are many good books that will give you great guidance, but you need to listen to your inner self, for if you feel uneasy when you are reading any of them, then it is probably not the book for you. When you find the right book with the right messages for you, then you will know from the powerful waves of joy that will fill you. Join a group of like-minded people and you will be able to see all the different methods that others have, and again you will find one or maybe more areas that you feel a rapport with. Also, you may find by just stilling your mind that your own talent will just appear and grow slowly or even quickly. This is what happened to our dear writer who suddenly became aware of voices within and accepted this as normal. This can happen to you!

You may only have one area that you can develop, but use this skill, for it is yours to use to stay in contact with your own angels and the many others you may like to call on. This is not a competition in which the one who has more abilities is better! This is definitely not so. You each have within you a developed area of contact that is necessary for you to use in your chosen way of helping earth and its people. Be aware we say, and you will go well in receiving your own personal messages.

Blessings are with you,
For I am,
Orchun

BARACHIEL 7/1/12

Welcome readers, for this is my first time of writing for you. We are going to discuss what it means to, "Go with God".

I am sure that you have heard this expression before. It is said as a goodbye to another. To say "Go with God", means that you wish for them to be safe and loved. We are going to look into the real meaning that was meant by this statement, for you who are reading this book of writings are of an enquiring mind, and this is the reason for our book to be written. All the information that you need to live and grow is in this book, and if you find one writing that is relevant to you then you can then look elsewhere to develop this are that as necessary for your growth.

Let us begin with the Word of the Lord, for it is His Word that has set the ground rules for all to follow. Indeed, it is the Word of God you follow, and with Jesus, it is for you to follow his life as this shows us that we never die. Do you think about the Ten Commandments that were read by Moses? I am sure that if you don't openly think about them, they are there in your mind and background of your life. Most religious groups have a set of rules that are very similar to each other, in fact if you look into these religions, regardless of which ones, there is a great similarity to the tales in them.

When man, with the ego in control, is able to lead a religion, the rules can be distorted and start to cause problems. I am explaining this because of the world situation, which as it stands is rather explosive. There are many rebels causing problems by trying to take what they have no right to and using violence, even against their own people. The true believers use these rules to follow what they believe and even if there is a parting of ways, they aim to live in peace.

God's Laws are well written for you and they are expressed in plain language so that all can comprehend what is meant by them. It is a small step from knowing the meaning of the words to actually following them. There are many who see themselves as righteous people but do not follow what is written as the way to live life. Let us use an example such as, "Love your neighbour as yourself". This appears to a simple thing, but as you look at your neighbourhood, can you say that you all respect each other? Respect is a good form of love, but at this time, neighbours rarely know each other.

What God wants you to do, is to live in peace and with respect, regardless of any differences of nature and way of life.

This is constantly an area that causes intense problems between suburban neighbours, as well as between the wider global population of earth. All who live on earth are children of God and are part of His family. Do you see how this Law of God is known but not followed by all, even though they feel that they are living a true, good way of life.

This is why, as you advance in this life and are closer to your ascension, that it is up to you to encourage understanding, respect and tolerance to all those who reside on earth. This is one of your chosen jobs that you undertook while waiting for birth into this life. Many of you fall into this category of helping to grow understanding by promoting the teaching of these other life styles and their cultures. As more souls learn what is important to these people, they need to learn to be patient and make space for the others needs. This is where all can go wrong if one tries to dominate the other. The need is to live in peace together.

So my friends show that you know God's Laws and promote them by living the Truth within them and slowly this movement will grow. Teach your children this way of living by God's Laws for the young are the future of the earth, and by doing this, you are contributing to your part by sharing the way to live the right life.

Do your part and all will be well for this New Age that has recently arrived, for God's Laws are the basis of it.

I am, my friends,
Barachiel

MAITREYA 14/1/12

This is about the story of what it would be like to, "Own the world, but lose your soul".

I am sure that you have heard this saying many times but did not stop to consider what it actually meant. We will then consider this together so that there is no misunderstanding. We begin with the idea of owning the world, which is not a really a possible thing to achieve. What you are doing in this instance is taking whatever you want without considering the concept properly. I am sure that you have seen these people who take whatever it is they want and then not make reparation to anyone. It becomes a greedy event of take and take, which does not include understanding the ramifications of what it is they are so crudely doing. Everything you have in life has a cost. Realize this and you are well on the way to understanding this area, as so many ignore this to the detriment of their soul's journey.

Let us look at this a little at a time starting with the cost of that which you want to own. Let us say that you can never really own anything in this world made by God, for He made it all for you to enjoy. When you pass back to Heaven, all that you enjoyed goes to another person. It may be your family home which is passed on to the members of your family or to a stranger who buys the house. The reality is, that you are only putting a deposit or lease on what you have to enable you to use God's gifts. Another saying that you will know is, "You can't take it with you", and everyone know that this is a real Truth of Life. You enter this life with nothing and you leave this life with nothing, so what goes between these two times of your life is only on loan for you to enjoy. If you do not use these objects properly then you will find that they will not remain yours for the pleasurable times of your life.

God gives to you with love, all that is destined to be in your life, and is very disappointed if you do not share the same with those you love. Then, it is very likely that at some time these joys will be removed from you and you will not receive them again until you understand that they are God's gifts for you to share. There is another scenario to this story, for if you abuse what you have been loaned then you may have this poor behaviour returned as karma into your next life or lives. This will be of the negative kind, and this is what you will be responsible for making for yourself, and it may take quite a lot of time to repay your misdeeds. You are the one who, between lives, decides what your own retaliation should be, for at this time you can see clearly that you have not used your gifts to help others to share and enjoy what it was that you had. Love means sharing with those who pass through your life, and until you do this, you will continue to live again in order to eventually understand.

Now let us look at another side of this tale for it is not a simple part of your life. The way of the greedy, for this is a very apt word, is not the way of God. These people who fit into this category are not the nicest people to interact with and we are sure you have all know someone like this. They take for themselves regardless of the end results such as harm, misery, and real distress in another's life. How do we get these people to understand for they are obviously not in touch with their soul's inner voice? Let them be and look upon them as the very poorest of the poor, for even though they may have the money to buy what they want, they will not get the true pleasure of the use of it, unlike the soul who is aware of the fact that they are in fact being given a gift from God.

Think of the joy that one will feel when it is shown to them that they are indeed receiving a gift from God. How can anything compare to this?

The greedy are normally full of bluff and false sense of power over others, and this shows that they are still very unaware of the true Meaning of Life. The best that you can do is to pray for them in their ignorance. It does not do any good to complain or point out their inadequacies, for they will not listen. By praying for them at this time, it could possibly end with this person picking up these vibrations and feeling a little guilty for taking what they do not really deserve. With a little luck, these persons may just remember, or have a little intuition, that will cause them to rethink their ways and remember to give thanks out into the world for their good life style.

Therefore you can help this issue with prayer and good thoughts, for when people take what they want and are without the knowledge that you have, your prayers can help this soul from returning for many lives while they are trying to learn this lesson of God as the giver,

Now you can see that you can indeed harm your soul for more of your lives by trying to own the world. All the world and its glories are free and God given, and all the material goods are given as a gift to you; a gift to help you have in full, the enjoyment of life that God wants for each of His children. This means all of you.

Blessings upon you, for you are all God's children.
Maitreya

ARGON 15/1/12

It is my great honour to be able to join the distinguished archangels and angels to write in this book that has all the guidance that you will need to live your life, for it is a handy book to refer to in times when you are struggling.

So to begin, I will speak of the things that interest me, and these are of course, helping you who are on earth. I wish to help you in your journey back Home to your Father in Heaven. There a myriad of ways that we angels can help you, for we know that not all people have the same journey at the same time. So we need to let you know that if you do not feel that a reading is for you, it probably isn't, and you will find your help in a different area of this book. This book is all about helping at any given level and with any with needs that you have.

Here then is my first item for your perusal and I hope that this will help you in the future of your life, when the future becomes your Now in time. I speak of the way in which you are being expected to live your life in one way by the majority, or even the minority of those who are in such a position to make rules. Many times you will feel that you do not agree about what is being implemented, and that you have no power to change these rules set in place by others who may not be of your level of advancement. Of course this will be difficult for you to accept, but what you can to do is a real problem.

There must be man-made rules on earth to keep the multitudes from causing problems such as anarchy and violence, for history has documented what a society without rules is like. It is impossible to live in safety this way. Through the ages, there have been many examples of this riotous way of life where all try to dominate, and the result is terrible fighting, death and severe misery for all. So rules must be made but you need to assess who is making them. With the availability of news reaching all over the world very quickly, you can look at these leaders as they set their rules, and as an advanced soul you will see what type of person they are. Are they being led by the rampant ego and doing all for their personal power, or are they deep thinking individuals who are really trying to make a better world for all? The answer of course is that the two types of people are involved but unfortunately the rules are often made by the egotistical leader.

Within a society that has freedom to choose their leader, your way of prompting the right way of life is to vote for this developed person.

If you have a vote, do note waste it or not use it, for even if you think there are no really honest candidates, vote for the policies that they put up front for their election. They do not stand alone, and within their Cabinet you will find some of the right people who can ensure that the promises made are not broken.

Where there is no democracy and instead a tyrant or military rule, then look at what is happening within these countries. These people are rising up against such controls, for they too can see the democracy and the use of free will that is in the rest of the world. They can see how they are being kept in poverty, and we know that your poor are wealthy in comparison to these poor souls. Of course, you need take into consideration those who rule from a corrupted religious base and claim that this is their duty to do so. No true religion in the world is against love, and encourages harming their fellow man. All faiths have a very similar background story and all true faiths have love for their fellow man as their basis. Any other regime is based on man-made assumptions and led by the ego, which causes havoc whenever in the position to control.

The Laws of the world were made by God and it is these Laws that you need to live by. Christians have their story of Moses reading out the Ten Commandments, and as I have said, the other faiths have similar statements, for it all comes from God. God made the world, not the persons who wish to rule for themselves and the accompanying power that they feel. This will take many lives of learning for them to eventually understand, but it will happen, for all on earth will eventually gain the realization of God, His world, and His Laws.

The answer then my friends, is to obey God's Laws, for all true societies laws are based on these great, all encompassing rules. They are the guidelines for you to live your life in an honest and fulfilling way, and the basis of all of them is love for yourself and your fellow man. For when you love, you care for and help others, and this is what God wants on this earth.

This way of life is coming, even if you doubted it at first, for you know now of the Golden Age that is starting during this life of yours. This is why you decided to live at this time of the world's history; you are to be a part of the movement forward. So with love and prayers, and showing the way you live, you are fulfilling your great plan and learning enough to travel on your Path Home to your heavenly Father.

I am,
Argon

VISHNU 16/1/12

In time, my friends, by following God's laws, you will all find your way back to your true Home with God.

Sometimes it may feel a difficult journey, but do believe that you all chose your own destiny so that you could learn the lessons that you knew were the next or final lessons in this, your life on earth. To understand what is that is happening in your life, you need to look with an open mind so you can see a trend which may give you an indication of what the lesson may be. You could also ask others in your life, for those who are close to you know you and why you are the person that you are.

Since you are reading these articles, it means that you are an advanced soul, but know within yourself that there are still other lessons to learn. Just think that if you know this, then you are well on the way to solve them and this will then open your life to further advancement. Within these readings will be an indication of what your problem is, and the way to solve it.

Let us start with what the problem may be, for all of earth's population has the same one to solve at some time or other. We will begin with that of not being able to accept others as your equal. You know that all men are made equal for they are all children of God, and this is so. You can see what appear to be many inequalities in the persons around in your life, and this is due to their individual level of advancement and to what degree their ego is in control of what they do. What you need to do is to remind yourself as to how all of the world's people originate, and to accept this. They are your brothers or sisters, and they deserve the respect due to those of your family who are struggling to grow. If they appear not to be growing, then accept that they will continue to return to earth until they have learnt this lesson. This then has nothing to do with you unless you are asked to help them! You are here to help them by modeling a life style or by actually teaching them if they are ready. Whatever way, you will be showing a patience that is necessary, that as a form of respect, is based on love for your fellow man.

There is another way of holding tight to your own life style and not sharing what has been given to you by God in His glory. This is a sin called greed, and it is cautioned against in one of the Ten Commandments. In fact, look at all the Commandments and see if you are using them as a guide to your own life. They were given as a guideline to your life and if you are able to integrate them in your life, then you are well on the way back Home. This does not mean that you must give away all that you have, but enjoy it and invite as many as are in your life to enjoy it with you. Sharing is much more pleasurable than doing something alone, and you will get so much pleasure from all the joys you have been given.

To master anything in your life, you need to look at the Commandments given by God and as read by Moses.

How simple this is to do, for it is spelled out clearly, and once you put these actions into play within your daily life they become a strong habit and you will be living the way you should. Without your belief in them, you will not be able to use them to solve your life's lesson.

Now it is your turn to go and look at the Laws that man was given. Read them and see how they fit into your life. Are you following some of them, and those you are not following, help you to start to find your problems? Once you find your way, you can think deeply and change your life slowly so that you are an example of the way God wants all to live. As you find the love for each other, which is the basis of all the rules, then you will receive great blessings from God and His angelic kingdom.

Your lessons are well in hand and you are on your Path Home, so you will find that life itself is a wonderful experience that you did not know about before. This is what you have been looking for in all of your past lives and have found in this particular life.

Do you see what it is you have to do now? Well then, take little steps. Take your first step in this life, for each life you choose will be different even if the same lesson is to be learned, and it is with your wisdom that you choose what sort of life you should live and the circumstances of it.

Blessings to you on your journey,
Vishnu

CONFUCIOUS 17/1/12

I want to tell you all of the way that you need to be within your soul to be accepted into Heaven for your final time.

This is a big topic but it will be simple for you to understand if you are close to your final life here on earth. Here then is what I will tell you, and hope that it helps you greatly on your journey. By this stage of your travelling we know that you are very close to finalizing all that you have had to do, but there are just a few things to attend to. Why you ask, did you say it was a big thing to talk about, when now you say that there are just a few things to care about? I will answer you. The total of what is needed within your life skills is quite daunting when looking from the very beginning. You know that you have passed a long way down your Path but you do not know specifically all that you have encompassed throughout your lives, and this is where the subject becomes one of enormity. This is easy to accept when you think of how many times you have lived for you to learn all that you innately know. For most of you do not remember even one past life, and certainly not what it was you were to learn from it. A few of you are able to regress in your mind's eye and see a little piece of a past life, but no one has the ability to see all their past lives and what was meant to be learnt from them.

In the last writing by Krishna, he referred you back to God's Commandments as a guide to all you have to learn, but when these are broken down into manageable pieces, each one can take many lives to learn. Then there are the lives of resting and testing what you have learned up to that point. What can cause some or many difficulties is that of your ego. This is one of the last areas that your need to conquer and we all know that the ego will not let go easily, for it has had you under control from your first life to this current one. This is where the complexity of learning lessons comes from.

Once you are aware of the role of your ego and see it as a dominating force that wants to rule you at all times, you then can work on controlling this aspect.

Do not think that this will be simple to do now that you are aware, for the ego will fight back and imitate the feelings and intuition that you have and so you will need to be very sure of what you are receiving, and then verify it with you guardian angels. You will receive their message in one way or another.

As you reach your time when you feel that you are not ego led, a feeling of calm will descend, but the ego can and will rise up again and so you need to remain aware of your thoughts and tendencies all the time. As you are well into this phrase, learn all you can and use God's Commandments as your guide. This is the time that you can see how far you have come and what needs to be worked on for your soul's sake. It is a time when learning is such a thrill since the knowledge that you are seeking will come to you easily, especially if you have asked your angels and God to help you find what it is that you need.

So I say unto you, take the time to understand all that you have learned and implement it into your relationships. This will show that you have reached and understand the final stage of love which is at the base of every aspect of your world. Love for all is what God wants you to give, and when you understand this, you will feel such an awakening of spiritual power within your soul. Your Spirit will speak to you and guide you. You will be showered with love from everywhere and you will show such love back to all in your world.

All these lives have been about developing yourself, growing in Spirit, and following God's words, for after your last life you will be able to live in Heaven and help all souls to grow and develop like you have.

By now you should be pretty sure of where you are in this life you live, or whether there is some more to learn and integrate into what you do on earth. What you are interested in as work or a hobby, may be just what you decided to do in Heaven before this life, so enjoy your learning and try other things that interest you.

For I am,
Confucious

ARGON 18/1/12

We will begin with the time that is coming, and this time is the Golden Age in which the world will shine and be as it should.

It is known that this will be a difficult transition, for as one looks around the world, it is easily seen that the world is far from what it should be. Also, if you look at the people of today, you can notice that there are many persons around who are aware and are doing all they can to help their fellow man. Awareness of others is becoming a part of life that all are seeing, even if the same philosophy is not shared. This philosophy is showing as a trend followed by the alternative life style persons similar to those who were young, about the nineteen seventies, who were called hippies. They were the first to talk of and use personal freedom of choice to decide not to go along with society's definitions of what was right or wrong.

Today, the way is being led, not by the religious groups, but by those who are interested in the metaphysical aspects of life and those who see that there is more to life than just surviving. They know they will live more than just one life, and they are here in this time to help the world in its struggles to advance. They know that there are such wondrous things available to those who seek them to learn what life is really about. This is a different slant to the way of old style religious teachings that gave you the story of God and His son Jesus, but in a strict way to control the followers. Today, if one opens their mind, they can see the messages within the Holy

Bible of the new way of life and thinking that is available. Most of this information is ignored due to the Bible being written so many years ago for a totally different world and way of life. Be aware my friend, for if you look in this wonderful book you will find the basis of this New Age life that we are all beginning. So both ways do integrate, but your mind needs to do its thinking out side of the traditional way.

Slowly this will happen because there are more advanced souls on earth at this time than ever before. If you are reading this book to advance your knowledge of this world, or trying to find your way through the maze of life and choices, you are one of those sent to help the world in its cleansing. This cleansing is very important for the world, for history shows that the direction of the world was lost in the ego ruled days of the quite recent past. At the moment the balance of the world is toward the negative side, but with all of the advanced persons in the world who are maturing now, the balance can and will be turned to the positive life that is promised in the Bible. These souls are emerging at a great rate and they know about the Secret of Life.

The Secret is that God is your Father and you are His child. He is always with you, and you never die as your Spirit travels onwards always.

They also know that God's Commandments were given as a guide for every person's life behavior, and when you follow them you will live your life fully and honestly. You will be on the true Path that takes you to your Home in Heaven. You are awakening at a fast rate and many are in, or approaching their last life before that wonderful trip Home.

What happens, you ask, when you arrive in your heavenly Home for the last time? You will find that Heaven is the example for life in the Golden Age, when it is fully installed on earth. All that you enjoyed on earth, and your skills, will still be part of your life. You may have a role as a teacher for an ability that you have mastered, a caring nature to look after others, or want to take your leaning to a higher level. You might decide for a while that you will explore this heavenly life and all that it can offer you. Where there were things that you were not able to do on earth due to your responsibilities, you will have plenty of time to do. After all, this is every ones idea of Heaven of how it should be. You will be able to use your free will with trust, for as you are not ego led, it cannot cause you any trouble.

For your next stage of life in Heaven, we will keep this story for other writings, for you will still be on a journey of development of self and the love that is all around.

Blessings,
For I am,
Argon

KRISHNA 19/1/12

I wish to inform all of the readers of the way of this time of life.

It is a different time to all others, for all times can be similar but different at the same time, and as discussed in a previous writing, this is why history is necessary. This is proven by going to the history books as they indicate a similar way of events in the past, but of course they will not be quite the same. All circumstances are different because of the different powers that exist at the different stages of the world, and all the levels of life development.

We will look at an instance that will show what it is meant to be. So far you are asking yourself, what is this all about? I can assure you that it will become clear and have relevance in your life while you are seeking the answers.

To begin with, let us look at the world as it was not that long ago. There are various cycles for those who inhabit the earth at different times, and there can be some areas that are the same, but also there will be some differences. Look at the age of the Victorian rule which is known for its very strict perceptions of behaviour, life style and thoughts. To see why this happened, let us look at the preceding time where morals were limited in their use, and when a lack of modesty and self control, along with personal financial riches made for a very free life style for those who could afford it. Though this wealth gave jobs to the needy working for the rich in their houses and estates, often these poor were not treated as equal in any way. Equality of men is God's Law, and this is love for your fellow man. So you can see, with the pendulum pointing to the negative side of life that the rich and their immoral ways were in control of the world's time during this era.

This became offset by the Victorian era which was drab, strict and with a modest way of life. There were some caring groups who started to work in hospitals and elsewhere for the poor, but of course there were still those who went on their selfish way. Here though, we are looking at the dominant trends of the times described.

After this time came wars and extreme poverty for the average person, and the work was hard and dirty for most of them. Working in the mines and factories was a great part of many lives, as was growing food for the population. After the First World War there was little relief, as the world went into a depression and into the Second World War. The free world won this war as they did the first, but at great expense to their countries. The world was poor and with great devastation needing to be mended. This provided work for those able to work after the war, and due to the war effort of women doing what were previously men's jobs, women were freed from house and children related duties to a degree, and became part of the paid work force. You can see that with the world free from war, except for a few countries, that all were able to work and the world mostly became a more financially stable community. Slowly, the improved financial positions of the average people began to give them a better life style, and the pendulum of life started to swing away from the severe aspects of the last era. Towards the end of the last century, the young began to rebel and pushed for a freedom of speech and way of life. This was the beginning of the New Age that has been spoken of; the prophesied time of equality, caring, love, and with the knowledge of God and the meaning for each life on earth.

Can you see how the past history has shaped what came after? By looking back, we can see that what will come is due to what occurred before. This is a reaction by the vibrations that were generated during these times.

By just looking at the last century and the Now of time, you can see that the free world is reacting to the thoughts and needs of its citizens and is changing for the better. The New Age will not come in instantly, as change is always slow, but this sets a strong base for what will be.

The future is not set in stone, not even by God, for you have a free will that was given to all at birth, to shape what will come.

There are so many these days who have experienced the many ways of life that exist, from being both rich or poor through their past lives, to the righteous and the immoral. These lessons of life have been learned over many life times, and so the positive power of right thinking is holding sway and growing as a force for the New Age.

A popular song of the Hippy era, told that the times were changing, and it is true. Use your knowledge of what has happened in the world's past to promote the positive methods that are available for all to use.

You are on earth at this time, in this life to do your part in promoting a free way of life based on caring for each other, for love is the lesson that you have to learn as the final way of life.

Blessings to you, for I am,
Krishna

ORCHUN 20/1/12

At this time of the year there is a feeling that Christmas and all its joy has passed and all that is left is work and little play. Do you relate to this? This must mean that you do not enjoy the work that you do, and this is sad for you. You are on this earth to enjoy yourself as much as is possible. Life is not meant to be boring, for if it is, then you are not stimulated to grow and develop.

Let us look at the way that you should live and how you can enjoy yourself, for there are two ways available. One is to leave your job, for if it is stressing you so that you can't enjoy yourself, then this situation must be intolerable to you. The other is to look at what you do and how you react to different situations and different people that you mix with each day. Do you feel that you are involved in some type of karmic retribution with a certain person, or do you not find any stimulation in the type of work that you are employed for? If you feel that you have done all that you can to improve a relationship in your work area and it is not improving, maybe this is a lesson for you to show respect for this person. Otherwise, you need to understand that there are some who are still very undeveloped and run by their dominant ego. We know that you will have tried all different ways to help improve the situation, but this is not always going to work with such persons. Think about how you can still enjoy your life in this situation.

The first thing that you need to understand is that life becomes more interesting if you look forward to doing an activity that you really enjoy. Anticipation of an event can elevate your vibrations, so that when you arrive at your chosen site, you are more than half way to enjoying it. You can forget the stress of normal days and this will be a great relief for your mind and body. Take time from your week to do something that you really enjoy, and plan for family and friend time too. What you do does not need to be elaborate but it should be simple fun, for sometimes this simple activity can grow into a great event to remember. When you remember the fun times, it stimulates your good vibrations and lifts you out of a dreary time you may be having. This is when you should start planning another fun event as this will help keep you mentally alert. If you are able, put some photos of the fun times and your family and friends around, and as others can see what you enjoy doing, you may just strike a chord with another at work which may bring you closer to them.

This is all very simplistically put, but for solving boredom and animosity at work you will need to start to respect yourself and give yourself some fun times. Self love is a necessary part of what is needed for you to grow and for you to be aware that others, regardless of their attitude, need respect. You do not need to like all the people, but you need to respect and accept them as God's child, the same as you are.

The ideas that we are giving you are to take your focus off the things that you need to do such as earn a living, and then put it back into the things that you really enjoy doing.

You can have the life style that you want by praying to God and His angels, for if this work situation that you are in is not set as part of your life plan, it need not be. You can think about what work you really would like to do and then ask for help from above. You will know when your prayers are being answered. Your dream job will emerge possibly in a way very different to what you expected, but you need to help by looking about, studying and talking to those in the type of job that you want. When this happens, do not forget to plan for your recreation, because relaxing is necessary to balance your life and body.

Prayer was given to you to use to ask for what you want, just as a child asks its parent. You are also asking your parent God, and both your earthly parents, and your heavenly Father, want you to have whatever makes you happy. Life is not meant to be hard or stressful for you at this advanced stage, so use little steps to plan fun times, and also to plan another career to support your family and have the life style that you want.

Change what you want to in your life, but make your love for yourself and others a part of this too.

You will be amazed as you will slowly begin to enjoy what you do every day of the week, and the problems that come up will not seem such a major issue in your life. Think of recreation as re-creation, and this is what will happen to your life if you follow our simple ideas and turn them to steps on your Path Home.

I am,
Orchun

METATRON 22/1/12

Today we will begin with the trials of the earth as it moves onward and upward towards the new life that is coming.

This life is called the New Age and has already started. You see trauma and trouble in many places of this world, but to have a new world, this one needs to be cleaned up so that it can be renewed. The old and the new do not always work well together, and this is so for the coming era.

The ways of this New Age will be quite different to the old, for the new world will be much better placed to help all those who live on her. How can this be you ask? We will tell you. We tell of the old ways of living for oneself and family only and not caring for the wider populace. This was not the way in the past for all the towns, for some were small and depended on each other to survive, and this is where the word community came to be, for communal living was so necessary. In this new world, when it has reached the Age of Golden Light, that is to say, when God's Light will be felt shining on all, there will be a communal spirit between all of those who are on the earth at that time. You can see it beginning to happen now if you look at the disasters that have occurred in the world lately. People are coming out to help those involved in trauma, for there seems to have been no other time that is so turbulent. This of course does not relate to the World Wars, for they are considered a man-made problem of major dimensions, whereas what is happening now is of a nature based need to clean the world in preparation for what is on the way. The future, in its infinite detail cannot be told, for it is subject to man's free will, but the vibrations of man are lifting and carrying all towards a better way of life. Life in this world at the moment is not positive and therefore, it is of no use for what God has promised for the world. The world of God is told in His Prayer,

"Thy Kingdom come, Thy Will be done on earth as it is in Heaven".

So you see that God wants earth to be just the same as Heaven. We know that to go to Heaven you will need to respect and love yourself and your neighbours, just as God loves you. Can you imagine my friends, living in such a world where all are happy, industrious and without the stress of this world now? There would be no need for strangers to fear each other for they would respect each other's differences and similarities. The fight to have more money and goods than others will not be part of this new time, since all will look after each other. The focus for life will change from "me" to "us", and on helping each other to develop and learn God's way. It will be much easier than the journey that you have made, for each step has not always been easy trying to find the lost the ideas that you were born with, and what your skills are. Some have fought long and hard to become good people, but they are minimized by another's ego which is out of control within a body of God's child, and God's child is what you are.

Let us give you a glimpse of life in Heaven for this is what you are helping to create in this life. You were chosen specially and agreed to do your best with your abilities. Heaven is a place full of Light and higher vibrations, and are more vivid than any one of the brightest days that you can remember. All are working together and enjoying their interests, and love abounds. Life is an absolute pleasure and is enjoyed regardless of what you do. You can involve yourself in areas that you have only heard of on earth, and the sights that you find will be wondrous beyond belief. This gives just a small indication of how life is meant to be in the future of the earth, and with your help and knowledge of how life should be lived, it has a great chance of becoming real. Only negativity can slow down the process, but with the people of today turning to each other and helping out when trouble happens, the balance of the world's pendulum is swinging over to a better way of life for all.

You see, man's free will cannot be interfered with, but the situation of this New Age will help dismiss the negativity that has been in this world for too long. Are you ready to do your work to help the world? You chose this work before this life that you were born into, and you were chosen for your development of faith and life style. Now is the time to implement all you feel within you. Of course, all of you have different roles to play and some are more physically involved, while others of you are showing the right way to work, live and love your neighbours as you do yourself.

It is your doing that this world is moving on positively, so enjoy your role for you are not alone, for God and His angels are with you always. Just ask them.

I am yours to help,
Metatron

ORCHUN 23/1/12

Hullo to all our friends on this day that is so glorious.

Why is it so glorious? It was made by God and His helpers for you to enjoy. Today we will speak of many things that are wonders on this earth but are not appreciated by all. Of course there are those among you who will say that you do appreciate it all, but are you in the majority? We will see if you are.

If you have had the ability to travel around the world or just to certain spots, then you will be aware of the many hi-lights that the world possesses. If you have stayed in your own area, then you probably have not seen what is around you, for familiarity breeds a contempt and not the wide vision that is required. Look around and see the myriad of things in your area of life such as parks, beaches, deserts, hills and towns. You have grown up with some of these and you take them for granted, and this is quite normal. Some places you have seen in books and on television, and you have been interested in them, but those who live there do not look at these wonders as you do. They too have grown used to their back yard as you have to yours. It doesn't take much to change this short sightedness and this is what we are aiming for today with this writing.

Let us look at the time dimensions of the day and look at the different lighting that the world has at dawn, the morning freshness, in days of sun and of wind, and the grey days, and then at twilight as it comes creeping and turns into the darkness of night.

Even the nights have shades of difference, and add to this lighting that may be strategically placed for effect or just to illuminate the streets and buildings out of necessity. The moonlight can have a magnificent effect upon anything on earth, for it can be a sliver of a new moon or the brightness of the full moon, or the silvery light that it sheds through winter and spring as the plants grow. I know you have all seen photographs of different scenes with the different lighting achieved naturally of artificially, so look at your own area at different times of the day, in different seasons and in a differing moods, for a reflective mood will give you different results to when you are in a boisterous mood.

Let us take the ocean as an example. On a warm sunlit day, you will see the sea twinkling as the waves disturb the flatness of the water. The scene is said to look like fairy lights twinkling over a wide area. Now change the weather to a windy cold day with severe clouds around, and this will add to the impact of what you see. This same view is altered to show a different vision that you may not have noticed before. We can then change the same scene to a different time of the day, such as dawn rising out of the water on the horizon. At this time, the colours of the sun are muted on the water, and then they change to a greater depth as more sun appears in the sky. Alternatively, look at this scene as the sun slowly dips down behind the edge of the sea. The colours, though similar to the dawn, are much stronger in depth and variety, showing from orange, yellow, pink, purple and all hosts of shades between on the colour spectrum. People will travel for many days just to see this great happening and they may instead get a grey day of storms, lightening and winds. The effect upon their senses can be just as strong as the opposite picture that they came to see.

The world is showing off all its attributes for all to see, all the time.

You are not really aware of this process if it has been part of your life for a long time. Look through the eyes of a child seeing the scene for the first time, and they are amazed at what is there for them. The first time that they see rain and feel it makes a great impact on them, as does seeing lightning flashes in the dark sky, and the snow or hail falling to the ground. What a pity we don't keep this memory of special things we have seen, but we grow up and get busy in this world by trying to earn a living for our family. We think that for our holidays we will go where everything is different, but this need not be so. It takes money to travel, and all the arrangements can tire you before you even leave, so why go? Within a short area of your home are wondrous sights, even if you live in the city. A crowded city will give you different views such as the old or new buildings highlighted by different lights, and the characters of the people who walk the streets and live in the area. Watching is a great way of wakening the inner sight of what is about you. Even if you do live in the city, you can still be close enough to beaches, parks, hills or lakes, where beauty is so abundant.

Look around my friends, for beauty is everywhere and it is there for you to enjoy, but to truly see all the intricacies of colour and designs you need to stay aware and look at all there is as a matter of course. You will be truly in touch with your inner being when you recognize beauty where-ever you are in your world.

You now know the secret of enjoying all that God has given to you, enjoy it all.

Blessings to you,
Orchun

KRISHNA 25/1/12

This is the day to tell you of what will be at the time of Now, in the future. We do not know exactly, as you read in the writings before, since free will can change the outcomes, but we can take a guess. Some things change greatly and the effect can be enormous, but others are just minor details that are absorbed into the pattern that is growing. Since we can see a pattern taking shape, we can then make an educated guess as to what will be, and we ask those of you who are in touch with us to guide your focus and prayers to what is a preferred outlook. This is the reason that so many advanced souls are in this life at this one time. This will continue for many years, as we need you to show and lead others into the right way of thinking, acting and being.

You are a special group of helpers who gave your consent and good wishes to helping God and His angelic helpers to make the inroads for this New Age, which is arriving as we speak.

You have read about this wonderful word where all will be loved as they should and there will be care for all who need it. If you have ever been in an environment of love and inclusiveness for all, then you will know how incredible this feels emotionally, physically, and also mentally. Multiply this emotion many times more to be able to understand the joy that will be invasive throughout your world.

By reading this book, you are focusing on your way of life and what you need to do to stay on the right Path to God. The more you find yourself, the more aware you will be and show to others that your way of life is available for all, just as Jesus showed in his life. That was his choice to live the life he did and to show you that you are doing what he did, in your own way. No one is doing, or feeling, or acting the same as you are; you are unique to this world, for God made you perfect and as He wanted you to be. This perfection is within you, and you are growing daily towards this spiritual peak. You are showing to others that they are able to grow continuously as you are. Of course there will always be skeptics, but eventually, they too will be believers in the greatness of the Spirit within all of you. All on earth will follow the well trodden Path back to their Home in Heaven, so believe in what you are doing for it is God's work.

In this miraculous future that is talked about, all of you who are beginning this era will be praised as the leaders who started the wondrous movement to have life as a Heaven on earth. You have taken on this responsibility even if you don't outwardly remember it, but some of you may feel some inward intuition about what you are doing or want to do. You are all searching for more, regardless of what you know, and this is what holds you to your task.

Go to your job with great faith, honesty, and love, and you will achieve all that you have set out to do.

As always, if you feel alone or off your true way, you will always have your guardian angels there for support. You know that you are never alone in life, even if you feel so, but just remember to talk to them constantly about what you are doing, learning and feeling, and ask for help whenever you need it. This may not be forth coming instantly, but as always, ways will be put in place so that you are given a solution, a feeling of relief, or that the situation has changed for the better. Help always comes to those who ask, so believe and you will witness the Truth of what we say.

Dear friends, you are such a great part of the way of the future, and you are needed by God, His angels, and the future generations to live in their Now, as you are doing today. You have taken on important work and you are very blessed for doing so. Enjoy your work and you will blossom for all to see, and as you unite with others of the same mind, then your prayers together will gain so much positive strength. So the wheel of life will turn, gaining speed and taking many more souls with it onwards to Heaven.

Blessings to you,
Krishna

ARGON 26/1/12

Today I wish to speak of what it means to get involved with the happenings of the earth at this time, for it is a very important time for all.

It is a time of great tension in the world, for this time is coming to an end and the world is ridding itself of all that does not suit,. This includes wars, battles, hatred and many other negative things that you all know are prevalent at the moment. We will discuss some of them, but the answer to all will be the same. Let us begin with the problem of the war in Afghanistan, for this seems to be one of the areas that concern nearly every adult that lives. The battles that are occurring are vicious, and many good men have given their life in sacrifice to try and stop the battles that surround this area. Can you see that this problem does need to be attended to, for the New World cannot come in fully with this sort of hatred and brutality in existence? This trial in the world needs to be settled for once and for all, but it will not be an easy job. The area itself supports a difficult type of warfare to any other that has been in the past, except for the Vietnam style war where the enemy was well hidden in a country that was ideal for this type of conflict. Afghanistan too, is a land where attackers can be unnoticed. The allied troops are training those who are able to support the country, and many of the people who reside there are in dismay with what is happening. What is happening is not supporting the freedom of its people.

Some militant men are using this situation to gain great power in the hope of ruling the world. They have interpreted religious Laws that are re-written for their own satisfaction and resultant power, for they want to rule the world as soon as possible. This is an evil that needs to be stopped as soon as possible, but we fear that it will be a long process for it started so long ago and with little resistance from the free world. The free world now has to do more since the problem is at such a great strength. Yes, some of the leaders have gone but there are many more radical men ready to take the power for themselves. Beside this, we have the power of these men over their own people, and some have now joined and turned their hatred towards others of the free world. Those who oppose the tyrants are not able to stand up against them for they fear greatly for their safety and that of their family and friends.

We have often written in these exerts that Jesus was sent by God to show all how to live their lives, and if you look on his story you will see very similar actions happened around him and the people of Israel. They were persecuted for taxes and their lives made unbearable by Pontius Pilate and others, for poverty was rife and they were not able to stand against him and the servants of his cause. Later, after Jesus went to Heaven and returned to show that none ever die, he gained many followers who were also persecuted. The story of throwing the Christians to the lions is unimaginable in its cruelty, but it happened never the less. So these times have been echoed in history before, and the world and many of its people have come through to live in peace doing what they wish to do with their lives. Even in the free countries of the world at times there have been traumas and violence, and gradually the times changed and people took control of the situation as they slowly began access the type life that they preferred. It is now happening in countries that have been under dictatorship for many generations; the residents can see the way that the free live and will do all that they can to have that same right to a better life style.

These movements are preparing the world by cleansing that which is not suitable in the world of love, and freedom, and beauty that is coming. You have been told of what it is you need to do to help the world as it struggles to rid itself of that which is against the Law of God. The negativity that this action of cleansing is giving to the world, needs to be replaced by positive affirmations and love for your fellow men who are suffering. We have explained that prayers are love based and hold many positive vibrations, and since there are more good souls in the world, when they pray for those who are involved, the rate of the vibrations will increase. Once a positive vibration is released, it continues to grow in intensity, as energy never dies, and it joins with other's positive vibrations coming from their prayers. Can you then imagine the positive strength that the earth has to wield over this negative situation within the world?

Yes, the world will win this time of trauma, for you have all been sent by your own wishes, to be involved in this sending out of all the love you can. Such trouble can never stand up against love. Love is all powerful, and since God has made you with a free will, it will be up to you to solve the world's dilemmas regardless of what they are.

You are ready, for the world needs you!

Help now, for this is the something that you have been looking for all your life. This is the link that you have been looking for, to serve your God and to make room for a brand new world, the New Age.

I am,
Argon

CONFUCIOUS 27/1/12

This is a time of growing awareness which is meant to be a secret in the world, but we know that this great mystery is not a mystery at all.

This is why you have all worked so hard through all of your lives, so that you could aim to develop yourself into a version of God Himself. When you were first in this world, you were very naive and not really aware of how to live life as it should be, so you lived very basically for food, shelter and any comfort that you could get. You have since travelled a long way, and your way of life is so much better now that you know about God and His Laws to use as a basis for right living. You now have guidelines to measure yourself by, and you also know by the feelings that you have had, that there must be more to life than just death. Many of you may just be starting to find out about your life, or you know what this "something" is. This means that you are on the Path Home to Heaven, where your long journey began all those lives ago. As you have read the stories that preceded this one, then you know that you are on this earth at this time to do a great service for the world and for God Himself. He is so grateful to the many of you who have undertaken this task, for due to the free will that He has bestowed upon you He cannot interfere in the world and its course, or what you do in your life time.

This scenario of a Golden Age was what God described to you and your angels, who together with you worked out what would be the best thing you could give back to the planet. You have so many talents by now, and so you chose what it was that you wanted to give back to this world that has nurtured you and held you for so long. It has all been your own choice, and the fact that you are actually doing this shows that you have held this memory in your heart all this life until you started to question what more you could do.

You are a very blessed person, and with your Spirit you are undertaking this preparation for the wonderful New Age that is coming.

This Age was foretold a long time ago in the Bible, and so the preparation was there, but volunteers were needed to come back for another life at the right time and do all they could to help. And so here you all are! You know of the traumas surrounding the world, and all natural events that are devastating for those involved while the land is cleaned and made ready for a better way of life. This then is your place in history! Pray for help for those involved, and send out feelings of love and care, for without this, the world will gain a momentum that is very negative and it will be difficult to dispel the force that it will gain. With the large group of advanced souls who are all helping and sending love and prayers into the atmosphere, the world will react positively and the momentum will be a force to take all that is good of this world into the future.

History shows us that miracles do happen and you are involved in creating a miracle of enormous strength. There will be no stress put on you, for the more confident you are in your approach, the easier the changes will be wrought. We have discussed this situation before, but it does not hurt to remind you that you are doing a valuable service for the mankind of Now and for mankind in the future. We do not look to what is to come but to what we are doing now, for Now is the most important time in your life and the world's life. Blessings are upon you, for the person that you are and for the job that you are doing, for it is no insignificant thing that you are involved with. Your descendants will know of what you have done, and they will praise you and be proud to be your descendants.

I am,
Confucious

CONFUCIOUS 3/2/12

Welcome my friends, for this is a great honour to be giving this message to all of you who are advanced souls. This is being done so that you can help this world enter the New Age that has started with such turmoil.

Do not worry about your responsibilities, for all you need to do is ask for help and you will receive it, and please know that you are never alone.

Let us begin with the way that you perceive that which is around you. Let me say what your thoughts are. There is violence and war, and a lot of "me", the ego, taking this world astray. The land and nature seem to be at odds with what you expect to be a New Age of beauty, of peace, and of love between all who exist on this new way of life.

This dear friends, is the cleansing.

The world is old and needs to be regenerated from the soil to the natural environment, and this is for all the animals and people who live after you. Yes, there are people suffering, but they volunteered for this life time so they can be a part of what is happening. Remember that everyone on earth, from the poorest to the richest, from the sickest to the healthiest, have chosen with their angels to experience this life today. You too, although you have no memory of choosing, can often feel that there is something waiting for you to do. This is a feeling that there must be something more to life, for if you feel that life has a special meaning for you, this goes back to what you have experienced and has occurred for you in past lives. Yes, the good and the bad were chosen and agreed to by you with your angels help. Remember that your angels are always there for you regardless of what happens. You are God's child, and as such, He has a parental depth of care for you and how you are developing. It is now time to do your "thing", as it is put these days. You are not alone and you have not taken more than you can handle, so pray for this world as it starts its birth pangs, for your positive energy is required to lift the world and it's processes to a higher level. With this, you too will be lifted higher and your Spirit will rejoice that you are entering into your original plan for your life, as well as developing your own self and abilities.

Confucious

CONFUCIOUS 4/2/12

We are here to tell you of what is happening and affecting the earth's future.

This troubled time that appears to be leading into a war torn future, is not a final result, but a variable of what can happen at this time, your Now. We can guess the future based on the events that are happening now, but it can be thankfully changed by you, and this is why so many of you who are very advanced souls, are on this earth now. Do you have a feeling of wondering, and that you know there is more for you to do in this life of yours? Do you feel that you have done all there is to do and that you are just marking time? Are you wondering and thinking of what you can do, and why you feel so strongly about this feeling of something more that can be done? Well my friends, there is most definitely a reason why you are here at this time, for you could have been born at any other time, but no, you and many like you, have volunteered to help this world into the New Age that has begun.

It is a time of trouble in many places of the world, and this is not a good sign for the future with some souls talking about signs that foretell of the end of the world. This does not need to be, as the world is in the throes of birthing this great New Age that has been talked of for many ages down through the years, and it is being written as history now. Enter into the story, the souls who are coming to the aid of this world of theirs, for you too are one of them. Without you and your prayers, the earth cannot enter this age without a dreadful struggle.

Nothing in life is pre-set by heaven or earth!

You all were given free will to live your life the way you wanted to. Yes, you will pay if you break the earthly rules which are set by people so that the world can be managed more easily, but God will not turn His back on you. He will be there for you when you call out to Him to help you. He will not interfere with your life style, but between this life and your last life, you agreed with God and His archangels to help this New Age develop and to help the with the problems of the world. What you have intuitively known is that there is another job for you to do! This is a great responsibility that you have taken on but please know that you are not alone. There are a great many of you with the same task set, but each of you will not do the same things. Some will be active in the trouble spots, others will be in back up areas, and some of you will say that you can't do these things. You have a support role, and this is such an important job to move the world in the right direction and give it strength to combat the negative vibrations that look as though they will overpower the good. Prayer, you can see, has been responsible for turning traumas into miracles throughout history, and this then is your special job, to pray for the safety of the world, the peace in the world and for the people who are taking this earth for their own domination. They need help most of all! This help is not to support the evil they are doing, but to turn them away from this side of life. With your prayers, God can step into the fray, and with His Great Will and ability, He can help you turn the world back to the right way and turn remove the negativity.

Are you ready dear friends, to do what you promised for God and His angel helpers?

You are needed now!

It is not such a great task to pray several times a day. No special words are needed to ask your guardian angels to help. Just talk naturally, and your words will turn into positive vibrations that will continue to grow until they overcome the negative attitude that pervades this world of yours. This is your time to help, and since you are all so advanced, you were specially asked to do this and then accepted by God. Go ahead and join together mentally and physically to achieve the birth of this Great New Age. The question you will ask is if you are you ready? We say the answer is yes! To begin, you will need to gather your thoughts and think about what you wish to say about the world so that it is phrased positively, for remember, you are sending good vibrations to help the world wherever it needs it. We have already stated that you do not need formal prayer but if this is your way then please do so. Talking within your mind is acceptable as is talking out aloud, but whatever way you do this, it will have the right outcome. Begin and voice your thoughts in a loving confident way since you know that what you are doing is done through love for your fellowman, and is backed with God's love for all of you. So you see that God is does not judge you, but He uses what you do to improve the world! His love is directing the world to a way that can improve the circumstances which are in the Now of your time.

You may be surprised to find that the people that you attract, and are interested in, are very similar in their intentions in wanting to help the world. You may find yourselves in groups who have the same knowledge that you do, and this too is ideal, for more positive vibrations can come forth and can be directed to where they are needed most. Imagine a group of twenty happy people in a hall and the vibrations that are generated are truly felt, but when the group becomes larger, the feeling that is generated is so much stronger and can often turn an unhappy person into enjoying what is occurring. This is what will happen if there are groups of advanced souls all asking for the same help at the same time. It is not easy to gather a group several times a day, and so, on your own you can still achieve the results that are needed as the energy goes into the area where you are living, and it grows as others thoughts and prayers join yours.

Can you see my dear friends, what you are capable of? What you can do in helping this earth reach its ability to grow into the fabled New Age of love and beauty, and equality? What a miracle you would be involved in, and as we have said, all miracles come from a plea from the heart. This is the dawn of the next world, and for your family's sake and your friends, and indeed for the world as it stands today, you can turn around what appears to be an impossible task. You are up to this! You are strong, determined and above all, an advanced soul who can teach the others around you of what is needed to fix this time in the world's history. Many are on their way to their final lives on earth and are learning their last lessons, for they too feel that there is something to do besides live in the world around them. They will join in with you, and the numbers of helpers plus their angels will accrue, and you don't need me to foretell the future outcome. The good vibrations will fill the areas that the prayers were sent from, and then spread into every space on this earth and overrule the negative vibrations that abound at this time. So, as the story ends my friends, we turn the request for help to you and yours, knowing that you have the boundless love to do all that this task needs.

I am,
Merlin

PARIS 17/2/12

My words may help those who are struggling with problems.

We will begin with the words of Master Jesus who said, "I am the Way". He gave his life as an example for you to copy, and though it may be so many years later, the same example works in this world of Now. All you need to do is follow the well known stories that abound and you will have the answer to whatever troubles you. Look to the renowned Saints and they will show you the way, for they have attained the life that Christ wants for all. Some may have been poor and down trodden, and many were not interested in the needs of the body, but instead focused on the needs of others. This is demonstrating great love for your fellow man, and the lesson to be learned at this time is to love and respect those on their journey as you are. Everything, animate or inanimate, is on a journey of progressiveness. Yes my friends, everything is part of God's world and made by Him for a reason. The fact that we don't realize about the inanimate objects of earth doesn't make it less so.

There is a lesson in this also, and this is that you need to look after this land of yours while it is still in your hands, for you are the custodians while you are on earth.

It is happening, for there is a growing respect for keeping the air clean and the water pure, and respecting the food produced by sharing it and not wasting what is grown, and allowing it to be shared. Be aware of the less fortunate countries and their citizens and realize they have needs that we can support. Before birth, they chose to live in this poverty for the need to know what it is like, and this gives you who are watching, the need to help. This is love for your fellow man, even if you do not know them personally. Do whatever you can to help for the slightest thing is accepted. If you are blessed with money, then donate to where ever you feel the need to do so, such as helping with children lives and their education, providing for water to be available and helping with food crops, and the teaching the skills necessary to make these people independent. If you are unable to provide the necessary cash or to go and train these people, then the road open to you, as always, is to pray. Heaven is awaiting your prayers so that they may start to help, for without your asking, the angels cannot do anything at all.

When you pray, you open many doors of waiting helpers and you lift the vibrations of the earth so that these souls can become involved with their own way of saving their part of the world. This method of praying has always been used by those who are in distress, but the end result is not often seen. The world needs your prayers at this time for it is struggling with violence, poverty and racial hatred, which shows as an enormous negativity within the world. At this moment, the feeling of negativity in the world is tangible to those sensitive enough to understand, and this feeling can spread quickly to others who do not understand but add their own negative vibrations to them.

The issue of finance in the world is like a web catching all the different countries in together, and the suffering economies are felt even by those who are relatively removed from this. Australia is part of this fear of what is happening to the world finances. The negative mood throughout the world is spreading through businesses, affecting people's spending and causing a major down turn. Spending is the way to help these areas, for all your money comes from God. You do not own anything on this earth, since all you have is on loan to you and you are a caretaker for the future generations. Spend your money confidently and wisely to help your country to recover and this will show the rest of the world how to manage their problems. You will not be left without, for what you give to the world is returned to you and yours. Give with love and respect, and the world will begin to prosper having learnt a very harsh lesson, that excessive greed causes great problems that must be faced later if not sooner. This is what is happening at the moment. The greed and need for power has caused this mess within God's earth, and this was done with the ego and free will working together. Pray to God now, for it is not too late to bring in the changes that the New Age needs so that all will see that God's Way is the only way. God's Way is what Jesus showed you so many years ago. There are many of you who are advanced souls in this world now, so join together in prayer and ask God and the archangels and all in Heaven to help.

You chose this time to return to earth with your advanced learning of how the world works. God is now calling you to do what you promised to do during this life you have. It is now up to you, for the reminder has been given.

God bless you, for it is you that the world and its people depend on at this time.

Blessings my friends,
Paris

VISHNU 18/2/12

Today it is my pleasure to introduce to you a good example of what life is all about.

Yes, you may say, this is about learning and love so that one can advance. There is so much more though my friends, for you have lived many times but know that there is more to learn. There has been no rush to learn and so each item you learned has taken many lives, and between them you have also had lives in which you were able to rest, use and enjoy that which you have learned.

Today we intend to help you with the subtler areas that you need to know. One of these is learning about the life that surrounds you, for it does have an effect on you and the way you live. Look at your acquaintances from work and see how you respond to them, and compare this to how you treat your family and friends. For many there will be a great gap between the ways you respond. You may feel that at work you should behave a certain way to your co-workers, especially if you are in charge and responsible for their work output. Have you heard that more flies are caught with honey than vinegar? This is true, and if you are not treating your workers with respect, then obviously they will not respond positively and you will not receive their best work. If their work is satisfactory, they may not give you any more than the basics needed, and if the time comes that you need their support for some reason, you will not gain it. In fact, your workers may indicate that you deserve what you get. You could also lose some of your best workers who feel that they deserve more positives for what they do, and be left with those who are unable to move on for whatever reason. This could all be due to your mental image of how you should treat certain sections of people around you. Look inward and see if any of this is part of your psyche. Be honest if you feel superior and act this way to others. It is possible that this attitude can be taken into your family life if you feel that you need to hold tightly to the control of those dearest to you. This is a lesson for you to learn, and this is that no one is in charge of another's life. You were born into this world as a single person and that is the way that you will remain.

All are equal in their life and remain so, regardless of what they are doing or not doing, to make it a success.

Remember that all are on a different part of their Path and at a different level of learning. No one is at precisely the same level of development or has exactly the same job to do while on earth, as they move forward and advance in the total sum of their journeys.

Remember dear friends, that if you treat your family, friends and acquaintances poorly, then you will lose the greatest joy there is on earth, and that is the love and support of those close to you.

This is not an easy task to stop and change your total mode of interacting, but with the desire to change, it can happen. Ask the ones who are closest to you and take their advice, for even though they may feel poorly treated, they are still with you through some past life connection and a respect called love. Let them speak freely to you and listen to their advice. Ask them to give you a sign that acts as a reminder to you if you go back to your old ways of interacting. Slowly you will integrate into your psyche, the right way of being with others, and the positivity of this will remove your negative behaviour. Of course your prayers for help will be answered, so listen to your intuitive self and also ask your angels to be with you and guide you to the right way of acting with others.

Life can be marvelous if you can adjust to giving out positive vibrations. Negativity will just attract more of the same, and you cannot have a happy life style in this way.

You are in this world to learn, and as an individual it is up to you assess your ways of doing and your results, for if you are not happy or satisfied, then look within to what may be the problem and work at it. You may be born as an individual but it is the world around you that you need to live in, and grow, and advance spiritually. It can be done, for you are not left to fight this battle of learning by yourself! Use with respect all that is in your life to better yourself, and keep advancing with the right motive to life and you will feel a sense of accomplishment that is wonderful to behold.

I am,
Vishnu

MAITREYA 19/2/12

Thank you my friends, for this is indeed an honour to talk to you through this medium.

We wish to talk further on the topic started before, for we feel that it is an important issue for you to understand. We are of course talking of the way you live your life and the effect it has on your journey Home to God your Father.

This time we will direct you to the way that is presenting itself to you and your reaction to it. This is about life and the people around you, for they affect you in what you do and how you react to them and the scene surrounding you. If you feel uneasy about this part of your life, then something is amiss, and by reading this you may be able to change what is your Now to a better one. You know that there is the history of what was and has now gone, and the future of which we can pray to bring in safely, which leaves only Now to live for. By living correctly and abiding by God's Laws, you are ensuring positive vibrations are emitted and that they will continue to grow as others follow in your footsteps.

Look around you and see if you are part of this positivity of life or are you seeking more? Are you disturbed by your surroundings and those in your life? All of you have a personal intuitive guidance system that lets you know if things are right or wrong, and you have the free will to listen or go your own way. It is your choice. What will you decide? There is a life of being aware of all that is, or a life of self indulgence which does not always satisfy, especially after continued self indulgence?

You have all heard of the very rich doing all types of wasteful things, and wondered as to why they are wasting their life when there could be so much more for them. These idle persons are usually portrayed as bored and self serving, and doing anything they want without much thought or conscience. If you see this with others, you can see it in your own life for there is a comparison that can be made. Have you worked hard for all that you wanted and now found that this does not satisfy you as you thought it would?

There is really only one way in your life that will give the satisfaction that all need, and that is of love, respect and happiness in what you do. If you think you have all there is for your life, then how can you experience the rest of life which you should be seeking?

The answer dear friends, is firstly to love yourself, for without this, how can anyone else like you.

So if you don't like the way you look or act, then stop and know that you are God's child! He made you to look this way and He only makes perfection. He loves you. How can you argue against this? He also gave you free will to choose what you want to do in life, but remember, it was between the last life you lived and this one that you decided on what it was you wanted to achieve now. Don't let the little things get in the way of the greatness that is available to you. Once you realize what you have chosen to do, the world will open up with such love and grace that you will know that this is the life you have chosen. The only thing is that it may take some searching to find what it is you need to do. Look around at the people you mix with and know that they are not just incidental to your life, but are there for a reason. Talk freely with them and try some of their interests to see what makes them content, and in this way you may just find one of them stirs up a long lost memory. You will find your place in this world and you will experience life as a joy, so it is well worth the search. Perhaps you have something that is pulling at you, so try it, for you are not committed to do this for all your life. You always have the free will to decide what to do!

Life, friends, is for living, loving, enjoying and having all that you want as long as no one is hurt in the gaining of it. Go and gain you soul's promise and enjoy all in your life, and you will advance further forward to your final life of training on this earth.

With blessings,
Maitreya

MERLIN 20/2/12

We wish to discuss what it is like to know the Truth of Life, and how to manage this knowledge.

To begin with, we assume that all of you reading this are part of the group who are familiar with the Truth of Life, but what are you doing with it? This is the next part of your journey of discovery to where you are actually going. The Truth is love and equality for all, and once you reach this level you will need to continue to show these values as being important in your life. Think deeply about this statement and assess your inner most feelings about showing others this type of respect and love. Do you respect all of those you meet? This is where the road can become a little blurry and a little bumpy, for when you look around, you can see others at very different levels and with very different characteristics that may in fact may be abhorrent to you. What to do? You know that all on earth are on their own journey and the mix is from the very advanced, to the new soul just starting out, and this is where it can be difficult for you to deal with. Just remember that at your stage of advanced development it is in your hands to show the way to others who are still unaware of why they are here. You have risen to the role of teacher, and though these new souls will not accept what you say about the way to live life, you can model for them and show them by your behaviour that you indeed have found the way to happiness and love. You do not have to physically show these persons that you love them, but what you need to do is to show respect to them for being God's child, just as you are, and so you are showing that they are your equal regardless of being in a different time of their development.

Love can be misconstrued as a physical and emotional feeling towards those closest to you, but this love we talk about is respect based. To respect another, you do not have to know them personally, but know of them existing in this world and accepting this premise.

The media shows you the people who deserve credit for what they have done or are doing for others. We know that you recognize them for their part in the process of life, and so a respect is born.

Respect is the aspect of love that you need to direct to others you meet or interact with.

This is what we talk of, of showing love to all, regardless of appearance and behaviour.

Yes, it is hard to respect those who are callous or brutal but you know that they are on a Path of finding themselves, so send them prayers to guide them and ask the angels to guide them to a better way of life. Remember that God and His heavenly angels do not judge you or them, but all judge them self and will change when the lesson is learnt. They will not always be like this as they will incur karma to balance the harm done to others, and then they choose their own karma with the help of their angels in between their lives. You have lived these lives though you have no memory of it, but when you are an advanced soul you will notice good or poor karma in what you are exposed to, just through living your life.

This journey that you are on is a wonderful trip and it should be enjoyed, for this is what life is about. Learning, extending yourself, and interacting with the whole gamut of life styles is what you are here for, and this is why it takes so many lives to reach the ultimate last life. This last life is all about love; the love for living, love for all in the world and enjoyment of the life you have and all you encounter as you travel on. If this is where you feel you are, then compassion for others is the way to show the love of God that is in you, so that others may see that there is more for them in life also.

So dear friends, be aware of others needs and tend to them where you can, and by doing this you are showing the love and respect for others on their own journey. You will be as a beacon in the night for others to follow and learn from. We bless you for what you are doing for your brothers and sisters of the world.

God is pleased and follows you with love and admiration for all you do in His name.

I am,
Merlin

ARCANE 21/2/12

This is the way of the people who are here to do so much for the world as it is today, for it is in dire need of help if all is to continue to work the way it should, and to support life for all who reside on her.

Let us begin with the time that is Now, for this is the only time that any one has. This time is in trouble, and those of you who have agreed to help have read a few writings that tell of what to do. Of course you have to feel the need to help, and then you have to decide what to do and what would be the best way for your skills to be utilized. So here you have two areas to think about, but there is more to consider. What talents come to mind for you, and when are you going to start the process of helping? Are you going to wait for others to join you or are you going to face this task alone? You can see that it is not a simple task you are involved in, but it can be quite complex.

The job at hand is to turn the negative vibrations to positive so that the earth will respond in a like way, and this is why you hear of so many enlightened souls being on earth at this time. There are more of these than at any other time in the history of the life of the world, and this is becoming a well known fact, but how can you fit together with others for the positive response needed, or do you want to go alone? This is a big question and it is for you to sort out. These readings are written to give you a guide, for many have prayed for help and guidance for the right direction.

Love and prayer are the two leading words.

You will find love within a group that is compatible for you, and if this group gives love to each other, the support grows for the job at hand and the vibrations rise and multiply. This is a little like the New Age that is struggling to begin, for this new world is described as a Heaven on earth with a life of divine love and happiness for all. This type of life will take some time to take hold but it will with your help. You cannot dictate what it will actually be like or how long this will take, but with your intention of helping and by showing your family and children who are growing up watching you and your good deeds, the number involved in this work will grow enormously. If you have two children and they have two children each, then the number of persons involved will be increasing at a great rate. Already, by looking at the number of births in the world, you can see that the world is expanding its numbers rapidly, but not all will have this life knowledge that you have. When they have your information, imagine what power you have to help in any way. These family groups will have great knowledge of what their job is on earth and this will cause a great lift in vibrations surrounding them and their area.

At this time, there are many families with large numbers of members sending many positive vibrations to Heaven. This will be joined with prayers for the cleansing of the earth as it is and a request for all to live a better safer life.

Love and prayers are part of the understanding of the advanced in this world, and you can grow this dedication by doing God and Heaven's work. Remember at all times that God made the world and all in it for you. He cannot make you do other than what you want to. If you want to waste this chance of serving, then He will accept that this is your choice and there will be no retributions given. Alternatively, if you want to help, then talk to God and become aware of the power which is within you and is guiding you to this advanced knowledge.

Yes friends, you have power within and without, and you are a very strong adversary for the bad and evil which is in and around the world today.

Inside, you have a spark of God's Spirit and it can be heard as it speaks and guides you forward. Many call this intuition, but it is your Spirit showing you the way and revealing the Universal Secrets that give you a power to do the right thing at all times. It is this Spirit that never dies, for it inhabits into new bodies which will suit the learning that the individual needs to grow spiritually until they reach their ascension. By this time of ascension, all have that which is necessary and can move onto other realms for more learning.

You never, ever, stop learning! That is what you were made for and have agreed to in each life you take on earth, and these tasks you willingly do once you are one of the enlightened ones.

You are one of these, for you have been given a job to help the world in any way possible and to teach the future generations how to help.

Be happy, give out love and prayers for positive change, and it will happen.

Love and blessings,
Arcane

BARACHIEL 22/2/12

We are well pleased as to the way that you are handling all that you have to do in this world, for it can sometimes be a difficult thing to fit everything into the time that you have.

You need time for amusing yourself also, for if you are able to enjoy your time, you will find that the work you need to do is not such a chore but has a sense of pleasure for achieving.

There are many who take life as a serious issue and they go about their chores as though their life depended on it, with the end result often of them being a stressed and possibly ill person. This is not how you should perceive life as it was not meant to be this way. God, as your Father, has the same feelings that you do towards your children when they come along, and that is of course, to indulge them and give them what makes them happy, He wants you to grow, develop, be well and be full of the joy of living. This phrase, "The joy of living", is not the chore of living, or the stress of living, but is all about happiness and pleasure in your life. While you are doing the job that you have chosen to give you and your family a living, then you should enjoy it. If you don't enjoy your life as it is, then why not? There are many positions in the world and so you do not need to stay in the one you have now. Are you depending on the work you have now because of difficult times and job losses? Then stay in your job and pray for guidance to find another place that will suit you more. There is no need to leave immediately, but do your research for a new job while you are asking God and His angels to help you.

If you ask, "Ye shall receive".

We know that you have heard these words, so believe and see what arrives for you. You will never doubt again or accept that which is second class or causing you misery. Turn your world into the wonderful place that it is by enjoying, being happy, and letting others feel the joy that is in and around you.

You do not want to live your life scraping together what you can for it will never satisfy you, and the resultant stress can be the dis-ease that you may have within your mind and body. When one area of your life goes wrong and feels so wrong, then nothing else will work properly for you as you go through life. You will find that others will turn away from you, including family members, for it is very difficult to be around a person with such low self concept and low vibrations. You are not in touch with your Spirit, which wants you to respond to all that is with joy and spontaneity. God and His angels are just waiting for you to say the words of, "Help me please", and slowly, with a new awareness, you will find that your life and attitude will change for the better. You can find a childlike enjoyment of even simple events as you go through each day. On difficult days there can still be some joy as you remember to ask for this heavenly help, and you will find your life will be transformed as if by miracle.

It does work, and it will work for you! Try it my friends! You have nothing to lose except your misery, stress and the disease that is building with in your system.

I am sending you blessings for your new life.
Barachiel

ORCHUN 23/2/12

This time of year is a wonderful time, for many are feeling the positive effect of the Christmas break and the nice weather in Australia. Take note of how you are feeling, and if it is a good feeling then remember that this is the way that you should feel all the time.

Feeling happy was referred to in the last writing, and how necessary this is for you to be what was predestined all those lives ago. Many of you have favourite times of the year, and if this time is summer, then enjoy it as much as you can. If it is not your special time, then what can you do to increase your pleasure? There are many hobbies that you can do while the days are longer and you have more time on your hands. Do not fill this extra time with work, for work and play must be balanced equally, especially if you do not like your work at this time. We referred to the way out of this problem in the last writing. While using some of your time to look for better ways to earn your living, go out and enjoy yourself with books, movies, or all the many electronic gadgets that are available for people of this time. You do not need to be out in the heat of the day, for certain hobbies can be done either inside or outside. The main point is to indulge yourself by making time for just you. Men and women should watch children through the day, for it takes very little to get them to start playing and making up fun where ever they are. They can enjoy a brick, some water and some dirt, and it can become one of the best things they feel they have done for a long time. Give them some paper and a pencil or glue, and the same thing happens. They are still using their imagination to make their pleasure. All you need to do to copy this, is to kick start your imagination. It will still work though it may be a bit rusty, but with use it will come back to you to give you the pleasure that is not fully in your life. Childish fun is what you need; the laughing, the activity, and with your mind focused on what feels good, is your way to go. With this type of fun you make memories that you look back on fondly and start to smile or laugh. Do this at stressful times! If you feel that the answer to a problem is not forth coming, stop, let go of the problem and start to look back at the fun ways and times. You will find that your imagination, now it has been stimulated and used, will start to give you more responsive answers to your problems.

Without fun you cannot be a good worker, for the active part of your mind is imagination and creativity, and that dies without being used all the time.

Creativity has given the world so many types of masterpieces. Look at the history of music, art, buildings, and the many other ways that men have expressed themselves without the tools that today's people have. Imagination shows that you can preserve your memories, and imagination is necessary for creativity. Where will you show your creativity? The greatest treasures are not created because the person had to work. Drudgery can never be the basis of great and memorable events. Creativity and self expression is where all originates. So dear friends, why struggle on when now you know the secret of beauty and joy in your life? Remember to ask for help if this way of finding yourself is difficult. You are never alone and your heavenly helpers want to see you having fun, especially your guardian angels. Give your Spirit within the space for some stimulation, and you will feel the benefit of this within your life.

My dear friends, our words are phrased simply so that all can understand, but the meaning behind these words is important. We are giving you guidelines for all that is happening in your life, and a way to solve some of your problems that you come across daily. We write as though the life you have should be just happiness, fun and going through life easily, but of course this is an ideal to aim for. Many of you do have problems with coping and existing with your life, but do not feel that you are a failure for not attaining a higher joy in life. What we write is to help your journey through life, by guiding, explaining, and telling you of the heavenly support that you have, if only you ask.

We are showing the way, bit by bit, to turn your life into an enjoyable event. Read, my friends, and you will understand.

I am,
Orchun

ST. GERMAIN 24/2/12

Well, here we are together for another of our discussions written for the benefit of those of you who are advanced souls. Our topic today is for the use of all who are not feeling as though they are advancing as quickly as they would like to.

Usually these people are either seeking perfection or are coping with some karma in their life. Either way, if this is you, do not feel that you are letting your life's promise down, for to aim for perfection is good, but accept the reality that this cannot be totally achieved in a life on earth. Yes, some of the martyrs you hear about seem to come pretty close to it, but in their own world and within their own character, they feel that they do not reach this ultimate pinnacle.

Let us look at your life dear friend and see where the problem is. Are you trying your best to rise to greatness now while you are still learning what the secrets of spiritual growth are?

While you live on this earth you will always be learning, for learning never stops and so you cannot reach this perfect stage that you dream of at this stage. This quest will continue for many more areas in your life even if you are going to Heaven for the final time at the end of this life. Many appear to think that this worldly life is all that there is to learn since it has taken you many lives, to reach the level that will allow you to go Home.

God has said that, "In my home there are many rooms", and you can take this to mean that life ends for the body but learning goes on for your soul on a new level. Here, you are finding out what your talents are and what you can do with them, for in Heaven there are many jobs waiting to be done. Look at all that is in this world and you will see the areas that need a helping hand. There are the forests and plants that need to be cared for, and animals to be protected. There are the children who pass over early and need some training for their next life chance. The people who return as aged, and weak or sick, need caring for, until they are able to resume the life's work that they have been training for. There are so many jobs to do, for you never stop developing and growing. If you did, what would be the purpose of all your lives on this earth? You are part of the big picture, as many say, for you are a part of God, His Plan, and His strategy, to continue to make the world a wonderful new vibrant place to be.

You know this as the New Age which is coming in as we speak. There is a lot of work to be done. I will not repeat what needs to be done as we have referred to this several time in our writings, but we do say that this is why you are here.

Not just for the perfection of yourself alone, but to send help over the world with the positive vibrations of change that are so desperately needed.

Can you see dear readers, that by seeking personal perfection you may be missing your true Path? Listen to your inner Spirit talk to you through your day and you will not go wrong, and then this will free you up to use your creativity. Within this part of your personality, you will be guided to the area that you enjoy most and therefore can help others on their journey.

Alternately, when karma is a problem, you will become aware of who is involved and what the problem is. Obviously, underneath this is a relationship or problem that you have had from other times in your many lives. Listen to the spark within you that speaks to you, or as you may call it, your intuition, to find out where the problem is. Is it you, or is it the others in your life? You both have been put together in this life to solve this to each of your satisfaction. Move towards a reconciliation of the problem so that you can start to enjoy life. If you have honestly done all you can to rectify a situation and it has not been reciprocated, then let go, knowing that it is now their problem to solve.

This is about knowing yourself and moving on, ever onwards, to learn your lessons and develop your creativeness to grow into the best person that you can be.

Do you see that you are not letting anyone down if you are not perfect? This is not your goal! Your aim is to be a well rounded, happy, loving and balanced person in touch with your inner Spirit. This is the way forward for you, my friends.

Enjoy your learning and the life that it gives you.

For I am,
St. Germain

MAITREYA 25/2/12

It is coming to our notice that there are those among you who are worried about the negative world that is in this moment.

There is a fear that it disasters may strike you and cause you untold misery. Do not fear my friends, for all that happens to you has been agreed to before this life. Many of you do not understand this, for why would you wish such trauma upon your life? You see that many have lost their homes and jobs, and if you are not in contact with the God's Plan you will feel resentment and fear, and dear friends, this is to be expected.

We will explain why you are involved in the world at this time. You are an advancing soul, and you may have requested that you return to this life to help and to show what can happen when people bond together to help each other. In the future this will be the norm, but at this time it is not a common thing for others to do. You will be aware of the cleansing of the earth, for most in this life have access to the media and the news reports coming in daily. The wars and the skirmishes for control of, and the intention of taking more of the world later, is normal daily news, as are the disasters of the natural kind that are sweeping countries as never before. The need of these people affected is great, and you will see that though the response to their plight is sometimes slow, there is a care pervading the world for those in need. You are part of this, for if you cannot give financially, you are sending thoughts of support for these souls.

Prayer is your way of support, for to pray is to send positive thoughts to Heaven and with this, God and His angels can help you.

This will address your problem of fear for all that is happening to you and your family, since the answer is the same. Asking for help can minimize the trauma and maximize the help given, for you will know that you are not facing this alone,. When you see an accident or are made aware of a trauma in the world, the first thing most call out is, "Oh God", and this is the first plea to help those involved.

You know that the world is cleansing itself for the New Age which is presenting itself Now. Before things can become better you will find that they normally become worse, for this is the pattern of life. Have you heard the saying that you have to hit the bottom, before you can start to climb up? This is applicable to many personal areas of your life. Look at alcoholics, for those who do make a recovery will tell you of an event where they felt such despair that it caused them to turn inward for strength to fight the habit. The same can be said of those who smoke and others with anger management problems, and in the many other areas in which you can see this documented. This is what the world is going through also, for it is cleansing itself so that it can regenerate into a wonderful new place for the future generations.

This is the New Age that has been prophesied for so many years, and we want you to be joyful about the part you are playing.

If you were to look back over the lives you have lived, you would find that learning does not happen as well if you choose the easy way out. It is true that you learn more from facing your problems than by not meeting them. This does not mean that your life should be filled with difficulty and stress, for we have written before that enjoyment of life in what you are doing is important.

It just means to be aware of the lessons you are learning. By using your intuition, you will know that the position that you find yourself in, especially if it is outside your comfort zone, is trying to tell you to solve this problem and thus move on in your life. Life is about advancing yourself so that you are aware of your spiritual self, and once you find this you will be able to advance confidently with any problem. You have then found the source of all that is good in your world, and you have become part of the Universal Force which can be used to build up positive vibrations to deal with the problems of the world. Do not fear for your life style, but instead prepare yourself if your Spirit voice tells you that you are in a vulnerable situation. You have free will to do whatever you feel needs to be done in tending to yourself, your family and their well being.

At this stage of your development you should think deeply about your spiritual voice within, and with your prayers, you will become part of the All Knowing, All Seeing, Universal Light of Life.

Your lesson for this life is to be a part of the greater Being and support it for the good of the future of the world and the New Age. Firstly, connect with your Spirit, and you will find that meditation is a good way to start your journey to achieving all we have spoken of. Work with pleasure for the promise of what is to come is a great incentive. Show those who are close to you what can be done with meditation. You can join a small or large group to experience this ability, or you can do it by yourself with the aid of numerous books, videos, and internet references, but start slowly. Do not become frustrated as this will make the effort more difficult. Just realize that this is a long term project which if you follow, it will give you great satisfaction in so many ways. The main one is being in touch with your Spirit and its guiding ability.

Try it my friends, for it will clear your mind of stress and fear, and open up a new way of thinking and acting.

I am,
Maitreya

MERLIN 26/2/12

There is a way of living that is not compatible with the way of life today.

This is the way of the "do-gooder", who takes it upon themselves to represent those who have an advanced soul. We are sure that you know that the person we mean is the one who is always taking over every plan or activity, and then tells you that they are doing it because no one else is able to. With this attitude are often the words that they don't want thanks, but then they go to great lengths to make sure that all know how much is done by their self sacrifice. Yes, it is wonderful that all who can are able to support people in need, but charity is a cold word when it is put out in everyone's face.

Charity is the word that can be used when people are giving of themselves in a quiet meaningful way.

These souls do not need thanks or praise, for they are giving of themselves for reasons other than recognition. They are giving out of love and concern for their fellow man! These are the true helpers of mankind and can do so much good, and they are not talking about themselves all the time. The other type of person has the opposite effect, as they are repulsing others who want to help in the true spirit of the word charity. Caring givers do not even think of what they are doing as charity but just do so out of the love and kindness in their hearts.

We feel that "giving" is the word that should be used instead of charity, for this word has been given a bad image by those who abuse this system. You will know about the groups who collect money for charitable works to be done. Some of these are small groups and some are large and unwieldy, and though many are honest with what they do, there are some who do not pass on the full benefit to those they collect for. This is excused by reason that there are "costs" involved, and then if they are investigated, it can be found that there are some persons involved taking huge wages as their due payment, leaving very little for those really in need.

Giving is generous! It wants no payment or reward!

The aim of giving is that it helps and makes life easier for those who need it at that time. We understand that raising money and donating money are two different things, but today there are very large organizations that coordinate the raising of money and getting it to where it does the most good. These companies, as we call them, are now being asked to reveal their income and show their donations to the needy. This information is available and so we say to you, stop and find out which companies give the majority of their income to the poor and needy, and those who keep their costs and personal incomes to a reasonable standard. This way you can be sure that what you give will get to those for whom it was raised.

The world at this time with its wars and disasters is causing a great influx of needy ones and this is increasing. People are feeling sorry for those involved and are donating more than they have ever done before. There is a growing awareness of the needs of others, for the world is turning from a "me" society to an "us" basis, and this is the beginning of the New Age which will be based on love for your fellow man. There are always those who take advantage of this type of situation, and so by your being aware of this downfall, you can support those groups who are showing the right aim for the correct result. Do not become negative about giving for this is not what needs to happen. Instead become aware and donate to where there is good work being achieved for those in need.

You are all here to support this new world in the making, and giving is your way of helping in this area. This is helping to renew the places which have to be cleaned away due to devastation and then rebuilt with new and better designed buildings. Other countries and towns are being devastated too, for though they may not be poverty ridden areas, they are built in such a place that there is an inherent danger for those living there. They too will be rebuilt and made stronger and better suited for their area and use.

Helping mankind doesn't mean financially only for there are so many ways to give a little of yourself to those who find themselves with some small or larger burden. Look in your own street and know these persons, for one day you may need them or you may see that they are in need of some simple courtesy such as a greeting. All in your world are God's children, and He desires that you care for each other at all times.

Show your love to all around you and others will copy. When one is helped then they will give to another, and so the cycle of giving, and caring, and loving will go the way it should always be.

For I am,
Merlin

VISHNU 27/2/12

"God be with you". We are about to discuss this statement.

You have all heard this statement said in many different ways. Some say it as a goodbye and others use it as a straight out blessing, but few put any thought into what it actually means. To begin with, let us look at it as a blessing, for it is used in conventional churches and others of a similar kind, so it obviously has great relevance to a matter regarding God Himself. When looked at in a literal way, how can you be with God when all of you are on earth? Obviously it means that God not a Being or Spirit far away from you who is just looking down on you. He is an integral part of your world! He is everywhere that you are and He is part of all you do every day.

Do you feel now that this puts a different perspective on the way that you live your life? It really should have some type of impact on you as you think of your daily life and what it entails. Would you be proud of yourself if you knew someone of greatness was watching you go about your business? Do not think for a moment that God takes the role of policing you or watching for any misdemeanors, for He does not. He watches you with love and hope as a true parent does with their own child. Remember that you are God's child now and forever and that He has been with you for all the times that you have lived. No matter what you have done in your lives, He has never turned away from you, for He watches to see that you are alright and hoping that you can see the folly of things that you do without thought. He will not judge you, but waits until you reach the time when you know that He is with you, and then He feels such joy that you too can feel it within your soul. He will not interfere with you as you go on your journey of living, but when you feel that you need to ask for help from Him, again He is overjoyed to be part of your life, supporting you and guiding you to the right Path for your life and the goal that you feel is within.

It is this time that you know that God is with you.
All is good, all is happiness and love abounds in your life!

You have reached the pinnacle of all your lives so do not lose this for material objects. God will give you all you want once you recognize Him, but do not arrogantly take or demand without some deep thoughts as to the way that it will affect you further into your life. It is possible to lose this treasured bond with God, but it will be you moving away from Him. He never forsakes you regardless of what you do or have done. He will forgive you if you go astray, but you need to forgive yourself first. You need to love yourself, and then be aware that you are on a learning journey with the last rule to learn, and this is to love all around you. Then you will find that you can love and respect yourself and all that you have been learning.

When this happens you are "Walking with God".

Walking with God will give you such a feeling of comfort and security while you go about your daily business. You are never alone, so if you are worried or concerned, do not dictate what you want to happen but give your problem with both hands to Him, for His ability is immense and He can see much more than you can. He will definitely solve your problem. If this does not happen immediately do not think that He has forsaken you. No, He is just waiting for a moment that suits what needs to be done. Remember that you are here to learn the lessons of life and what you're involved in may be one of those lessons. He will not abandon you so keep talking to Him to find the learning point, and then He, with you, can solve your problem.

When you say goodbye to anyone, remember that you are really saying, "God be with you". This is a shortened version of the words. If you were to use the full term then others may come to understand what this means. Imagine if the awareness of God was brought to the forefront of everyone's mind? Those who advancing quickly, will be able to use the knowledge that God is with them as a parent figure, guiding them along so they may have the best life possible and still learn their lessons. Life does not need be difficult, for with your hand in God's you can be helped as a child is by a caring parent. This is the great similarity between God as a parent and an earthly parent.

A parent should give their child security, care, and love, with lessons in life behaviours so that the children can make their way in the world. It is said by earth parents, that once you have children, you never stop caring for them and loving them and are always there for them regardless of how old they are. This you can see is God's way too. All He wants is to see you develop and enjoy your life while abiding by the principles that He set down in the Ten Commandments. These are His rules, just as all good functioning homes have guidelines to follow so that you know if you are achieving the right life style or not. It is this that shows you the way to gaining a pure soul.

God be with you,
I am,
Vishnu

ARGON 28/2/12

This time dear friends, I wish to discuss with you what can be done when you find yourself in a situation that is seemingly and annoyingly unsolvable. A situation in which you find that all you are reading does not cover adequately, regardless of which way you look. Some of our writings will appear to be very simplistic but life is not always like that, and so what else can you do to achieve a solution?

Of course you will say that there is prayer and that always works when you ask God for His help. We have told you many times that He will answer you. Your guardian angels too are there to ask, but sometimes you are in the middle of a learning time to see if you have learnt a past lesson, or are learning a new lesson. If you find yourself unsure, then what do you do in the immediate Now of the problem? Your problem will be solved at the time God deems right for you, but in the interim it can become difficult. Know that you are being tested, not in as school process, but to see if you have gained enough skills to deal with what is occurring in your life. The first thing you do is pray as you know that it will help you. To know this gives you a better self concept and some confidence in your own ability to do what you feel is right in the first instance of the situation. We have said before, that if you love yourself in the true way and not as a dominating ego, then you will be calm enough to continue for the time necessary.

With this confidence and the knowledge you have as an advanced person, you can then concentrate and ask your inner soul who knows all about your life to see what the problem is. That appears to be the easiest part for then you need to evaluate what has caused the problem. Is it a different type and style of person and their personality? Note this down, for this may be just the tip of the total. Can you see yourself within the behaviour of the persons involved? We ask this because often individuals find that they don't like in others that which is in them self, and this can then cause a strong adverse reaction to this person. This is the time to be honest with yourself, for if you are not, you will fail to solve this dilemma. It will be easier to glance at the overall picture if you have it written down in front of you and sectionalized to see if the same item is written more than once.

You can find that there can be many problems within the one, and so there is a need to address them all. What you are doing is making a picture of your interactions with others and then seeing if there is a particular time, or situation which causes the reactions to surge through you. What about if you are dealing with a less advanced person who is in the hands of their ego? What if you want to discuss what is happening each time you are together and they are still working at the ego level of blame for all, instead of being able to see the total screen as you have? All the talking in the world will not get through to a person such as this, so do not put the blame on them, for this is due to the developmental stage they are at. Therefore, it will be up to you to try and make a change happen. You need to be sure that a change for the better can occur, for if you enter this with a negative attitude, then it will not happen.

Many people you will notice, are creatures of habit and this is due to their ego. The ego's job from the start of your lives has been to train you in the way of looking after yourself. Compare this to a new baby that is quite helpless at first. The parents are the ones to do the caring and then the training of the child until they can look after themselves, just as the ego has done for you. You do reach a stage where you do not need your parents telling you what to do, and you can go into the world to make your own way.

The ego is like the parent who will not let go; the one who feels that they are and must be in control of all in your life.

Some souls are still bound by this ego which wants to dominate and others are at the stage that they are trying to loosen the shackles. The ego is not a reliable source of direction for you, for what the ego does is for its own good. You have seen those who are very egotistical, but one day they too will find the way to put their ego back to where it belongs for it has by then done its duty. It is now your Spirit's turn to show you the right way. This is the internal warning system that gives you intuitive messages, until you realize that this is your eternal Spirit which is guiding you to learn the correct lessons of life.

The ego based person has become a creature of habit and finds it hard to initiate any new behaviour, while the Spirit led person is willing to work through a problem. Conflicts in every area of life, and in all war ravaged countries are due to the ego led persons.

You can now see how big a problem this can be to one trying to find the answer! It is no one's fault, but it affects everyone. Since you are the advanced soul it will be up to you to change the situation, since the others won't and in fact can't.

If you have found that it is a personality problem, then you can try to have someone else interact with them as much as possible in the work place, and it should be easier in a social situation to interact away from these persons, as long as it is not to noticeable to them. By knowing what you are doing should avoid more stress in your life, and that in itself is a large step forward.

You are in control of your life, and with help from praying, you will solve the problem without much ado. You will have learned a good lesson to be used in any situation, and you can teach others how to act also.

Blessings upon you,
Argon

MAITREYA 29/2/12

I am glad to be with you again dear friends for I wish to tell you about what it is to be free.

Not all in the world are free, for there are those in the prisons and others who live under a regime of domination. There is another type of lack of freedom and many so called "free" people are under its domination. This is a self imposed lack of freedom in which they set rules for themselves. These rules are extra to the boundaries of normal government rules which are set for the society to exist peacefully and safely.

We will look at this issue that so many have caught themselves in, and where it comes from. Firstly, the rules they set can be due to the family in which they grew up, and this may be where they have not been exposed to a free life where this tightly connected set of rules is not used. Like usually attracts like, and some of these rules are set within the framework of a so called "religious institution" or a similar group. Many of these have been set up to make money from the naïve and unsuspecting, and to do this, the rules are that are set keep them away from seeing the real world and comparing it with how they live. Alternative life styles often have the same input as to ruling those who are seeking a different life. Regardless of the reason, these souls are not free from such extreme ideas for their way of life. As they mature, they may find the habits of their youth ingrained and continue along the same rigid path as their parents did.

This need not be, for all it takes is a person to start thinking about what is in their life and to feel that this is not the way of true happiness. Happiness is what everyone wants in their life and if it is not part of your time, then questions will need to be asked. They will start in the mind, and then find a way to be spoken aloud to them self or to another that they find are feeling the same way. Once this happens, the Spirit is finding its way to lead you to freedom.

Freedom is living to the basic rules of the Ten Commandments that God gave to Moses.

The other societal rules are to ensure that the cities and countries are run well but not in a restrictive way, for most of the rules in the advanced countries are just. The restrictive groups do obey the laws set down by society to the greater part, for they must obey the law or pay the penalty. Where they go wrong is by diverging and using their own interpretation of God's Laws, and implementing their own ideas. Normally this is a means to control others for their ego is rampant within them. There is little true love expressed as in a spiritual way, for with love, all are free to help others.

Being free means giving to family, friends, acquaintances and others who live in the world, and in particular to yourself. It is doing what you feel is right by learning to develop your abilities and knowledge so that you may serve God. What a wonderful time you will have during this life, and you will shine as an example of the freedom that has been given to you by God Himself. All on earth have this freedom too, but we just need to show those who are lost in others domination.

Freedom was and still is every ones right.

If God Himself will not interfere with what you do until you ask Him, what right has anyone else have to rule another and take their freedom? No one my dear friends, so the work ahead for many of you is to open the eyes of those who are close to being able to use their own spiritual self as a guide. This is not an easy job to do and you need to be aware that by helping one to understand, you do not over step their right of choice. What you can do is to answer the questions that will come, with love and patience. Remember that they are struggling with a new concept and it will take some time for them to adjust to such ideas of freedom. Put yourself in the place of a teacher who is teaching a new subject and who needs to keep reviewing the subject until the student's mind has accepted it. You have a great amount of information at your finger tips, in books, papers, technology and the media, so use any or all the methods when you are asked if you can support what you say.

Freedom is for everyone so enjoy it but do not feel you have to struggle with any problems by yourself, for you are never alone. God is always with you, but you still have the freedom to do what you want with your life.

Teach others and enjoy your life. You are definitely free to do so.

I am,
Maitreya

ORCHUN 1/3/12

The time has come to be aware of the day of darkness that has been prophesied since life began. It is said to be arriving in December this year of 2012, but do not fear dear friends, for it will not be as has been said, the ending of the world!

This will not be!

This day came into the knowledge of man as the end of time because the Mayan calendar ended on this day. The Mayans ended their way of measuring time on this date as they could not perceive of life going any longer. The Mayan age was an exceptionally long time ago, and it was impossible for them to understand such an enormous amount time passing in life so they left the calendar at a that date. Others have also taken the ending of this written calendar as the end of the world too. It is being written in books and magazines and other media, and the information is now open to those who have not reached an advanced state of learning through their earthly life, and they are open to the fear factor of the unknown. Nostradamus had a talent for seeing the future but he was still an earth based man who could take the signs he received and interpret them wrongly. Many of his writings can be interpreted in different ways due to the inherent perceptions of the reader.

There have been many psychics in the world of differing abilities, but all of them, including today's best clairvoyants, are still souls who are earth bound, and the information they receive needs to be filtered through this earthly layer and their life understanding. Thus they are open to interpreting what they hear, and this is where the person's own views and slant on life can be mixed with the messages they receive. In the books that cite Nostradamus' works, many state this fact, but those reading do not understand the subtle difference that a description can make. Choose words to describe that which you are unsure of or have not seen and another will put their own understanding to this based on their own life experiences. Some of his readings can be related to events that have happened in the recent world events such as the destruction of the two towers in New York, which is known as the 9/11 event in America. Other writings are very ambiguous and so are available for different interpretations, and this is why it is said that some of his prophesies appear to be wrong. This is usually said by those who do not understand the ability that is available to all who are able to reach their inner Spirit.

Your Spirit knows all that was in the past and all that could be possible in the future. Remember that the future is not set in "concrete" but is open to those of the earth who through their free will can change it.

So, dear friends, do not be afraid of something that was foretold so long ago when those on earth had no idea of the great differences and advancements that have been made. They made their decisions affecting their life based on the conditions around at that time, but they do not affect today. If you are still worried then ask for support and pray, for God and His angels are just waiting and will support you in your needs.

Life as we said has changed greatly and the end of the world that has been forecast before by many, but it has always come and gone, and you continue to live on and grow. This December day will be the same for otherwise the New Age that has begun will not come through as prophesied. These two prophecies are at odds with each other, for there cannot be the end of the world and the continuance of the New Age.

This Age has started already, and is showing signs by many advanced souls who are following God and working for a new way to live in peace and love.

Ask yourself, how can this be happening if the world is going to end this year?

Yes, there has been grave fighting and there have natural disasters all over the world, but this is just the earth cleansing itself. It is preparing a new canvass for the future to be painted on.

All is good, for the world will continue for many millenniums to come. Pray for this New Age, for your family members will receive the benefits of this wonderful world that we are dreaming of.

For I am,
Orchun

ARGON 2/3/12

Let me tell you of what could be in the future even though this is not set, for the free will of man comes into the equation.

Of course we are talking about the New Age. This is a time that has been spoken of for many years and now has started. It is a tentative start, but the expectation of what has been written gives those involved a lift, for the waiting is over. The transition has begun.

We have written often about the cleansing of the world as is happening now, but it is of such great proportions that many fear the future. Do not fear my friends, for you are not sent any more that you can cope with.

All will be well, as a feeling of needing to help each other is beginning to pervade the world, and this is the start of love for your earthly brothers and sisters. Can you see that kindness to each other is indeed a step forward from the self-centered lives that many persons are living? The focus has been on the ego which takes but will not give back. We are now moving forward with great blessings upon you.

Today we will look at the strong possibilities that are due to come into the world as it travels on. For a start, we note that people will be more caring towards each other, and of course this is one of God's requests that you "Love others as you love yourself". When love is to the forefront, life is definitely more enjoyable, Love makes those who have found it, happier and more accepting of what is happening around them. This makes everything that you need to do less stressful,l and this is definitely needed in life as it is today.

Love is the key word for life, for it is one of the final lessons that you on earth to learn.

God is all about love and He wants your life to be about love too, for He, as your heavenly Father, wants you to be happy at all times.

One of the next changes you will find is that of sharing all the material goods that you gather around. Not just sharing with your family but with those who live in the world around you. This does not mean that you will give all that you have to any one, for this will not work, but sharing them with your larger group of acquaintances is what will happen. This sharing will be a source of joy, not only for others involved, but also for you, for happiness is catching. When you go into a room of happy people it is very hard to remain stressed or cross. Happiness is catching especially when in a larger group, for the vibrations that they emit are positive and they invade others' auras. This is what a party does for one of any age. The results for those involved are clear to see.

We will find the New Age will be full of love, happiness and sharing. What a wonderful direction this planet is heading and what a wonderful life for those involved, and these souls will be your descendants. You are going to have an impact on your own family and their lives, and those of their children and then their children. Each generation will move further forward into the Light that love brings.

There will other changes involved, such as the way that a living can be gained to support families, for work will still be necessary. Traditional jobs will go and replaced by others that are now in the making. Shops will change as technology becomes deeply engrained in society. It is showing now as sales are happening on the internet with increasing participation. Buyers will be able to stay home or at their place of work to see what is available, and then compare the prices. This is already cutting down the number of persons going to the shops, and so these old ways of life will also need to change to continue on. Work will be based on a person's needs such as time available to work, the days they want to work and the skills that they want to learn. At the moment it is the owners and managers of the businesses who tell the workers what to do and the result is not always good for the staff, so they often show their unhappiness by not giving all they can to the position. There are better ways coming to run businesses so that all involved will gain prestige and a positive self concept, and the business will of course thrive.

There are so many ways this old word will improve, for if we look at the environment and see the amount of rubbish being left around, harming nature and the animals and this is not a positive aspect of the world. In the future when it becomes the Now in your time, more will be using recycling for most rubbish, and ways will be found that are better to get rid of the rest. Care of animals of all kinds will improve, especially for the food animals. At this moment they are slain in a non humane way for the main and this needs to change. Animals have been given to the world to feed the population, but the need is to have the animals treated humanely so they do not endure the fear that they do now. This feeling of fear pervades the flesh that you are eating and is not good for your health. There will be alternative ways of eating and many more will try vegetarianism or being vegan. Plants also feel pain when picked but they were made for this as their role to help feed the world. The world of plants will have more respect given it and this will be well deserved, for they accomplish much for the humans and animals. Think what life would be without plants of all the types available? No wonderful gardens, and forests, or backyard vegetable gardens, and no farms to provide vegetables for the shops to sell. Without nature and people supporting the life of plants, the world would not continue and neither would the human race as you need the food and the oxygen that plants provide. Natural products and growing methods will be introduced so that poisons are totally eliminated, for it is accepted that they are a danger to the health of all on earth. Already you can see many illnesses of the body that are related to the poisons in the foods that are eaten and more will arise if changes are not made. These changes will happen in the New Age.

Finally, the babes that will be born into this world will be more advanced than ever before.

You can see this is happening now, for the young seem to know how to use the new technology that abounds. They will have specialized information within them ready to use in the world that is coming and their children will be even more adept for the world they are entering.

Dear friends, look to the Now of your life and begin to set the changes that you feel are right for the world and you will be doing a great service, for this is the responsibility you have taken on in this life. Set the future through the Now of your life, and the world of your descendants will be a wonderful caring one for all to live, and love, and enjoy.

I am,
Argon

MERLIN 5/3/12

Welcome my dear friends, for today we wish to speak of the ways you can free yourself from the dreary responsibilities of life.

This is difficult you reply, but really this is just a point of view that needs to be altered. We will begin. We will look at what appears to be the normal type of life that is lived in your part of the world. Of course, this does not fit every-one's life which can be influenced by other events. We re-iterate that this is to be taken as the seemingly average way to live which includes going to work, caring for a family and its needs and dealing with the lack of time and stress this brings to you. There seems to be no way to fit all you have to do and what you want to do into the day and this brings the stress aspect into your life. Once you become stressed your problems becomes more difficult and more intense as you feel that you are under a great weight that is smothering you. With this, you find that the person you were in the earlier part of your life has just about gone and is replaced by a shadow of your former self. This then can lead to family relationship problems, and even the breakup of the family unit which in turn causes more stress in your life. How to cope is the problem, and how to get from under the great load on your shoulders is what you have to find. Look around at the society that you live in and you will see that so many of your peers are in the same predicament. It is not just your problem but it is a major one facing so many today. To adjust your life is not easy but you do have the incentive to do so, for living the way that you do is causing you severe unhappiness and preventing you from enjoying your life. More than this, stress will cause illness and diseases to make your life more difficult, and this is not acceptable to you.

We will start at the beginning with what you want in your life changed. This needs to be the foremost thought in your mind. This thought needs to be desired more than you have wanted any other thing in your life up to now! You will need to tend to the ways that can fix your problem as you would care for a new born babe. This is not an extreme statement, for when you are in the midst of a life crisis, all your resolve is under attack from outside demands. When you really want to change your life, you can do it. Think how far you have come since you were a child preparing for life and look at what you have achieved, for you are maintaining yourself and most likely a family, and this is a great feat in itself. You have done this with your free will and determination, and so these are indications that you can change your life so you may enjoy all of the benefits that you worked so hard to gain.

The first thing is to realize that you are not alone in this venture. You should know now from these writings that God is always with you, and so are your angel guides and any other angels that you desire. They are there to help you in any way, for this is their role. As well, you can bring your partner into the equation, for they too may be feeling the same as you about their life in the work force and at home. It is said that a problem shared is a problem halved and this is the best way to approach your journey to a better life. So at this early stage you have heavenly support and family support. You now need to find a starting point that suits you so that other changes will be able to be slotted in after. Even one change will be like a breath of fresh air in your way of life. The best way is to take some time for yourself. I hear you say that there is no time available and this is where all your problems started! We suggest that by making a list of what you do on your weekends, you are sure to find some things that can be left.

The idea behind this whole writing is to learn to delegate and manage your time.

Do not do all and be all, for this is your ego in control.

Your ego wants you to think that all in your world rests on your shoulders, and we say firmly to you that it does not. If you were to leave the work that you to do and move on, then yes, you may be missed for a short time, but soon someone else will be doing want you did. No one is irreplaceable and no one needs to sacrifice themselves for work. Can you see that the thought of wanting to be needed is driving you and this leads to doing more than is necessary?

You are seeking outside gratification for your work, rather than having the necessary self respect and self love that will tell you that you are doing well.

If you accept that you are doing your best, then that is all the recommendation you need. Look and see if your other work mates are letting you do some of their work too, for this can happen. Delegate the work that is not yours and which should be done by another, and that which you can return to them without loading them unfairly. If you interact with courtesy and respect to those you work with, then you will mostly find it is returned. Do the same at home, as not everything needs to be done by you. Some can be left or delegated for a few dollars to someone else such as your children, or someone with the time to care for all that is needed to keep a home going. Delegate is the word for you to learn to use.

On the weekends take some time to indulge in the areas that you enjoy such as gardening, talking to the neighbours, going for a walk or taking a trip in your local environment. This will feel like a mini holiday, for another saying is that is true is that, "a change is as good as a holiday". You should return to work refreshed as long as you have been able to squash the thoughts of not doing, and accept relaxing instead. This would be your ego trying to make you feel guilty about giving yourself some enjoyment, so ignore it. It is God's wish that you enjoy the life He has given you. Listen to your inner self telling you that you are having fun and that it feels good, and ignore the voice that is demanding that the world will stop if you do not work all the minutes that are in your life.

This is the attitude that you need to muster; the attitude is that you love and respect yourself, and know that God is telling you to relax and enjoy by delegating some of your responsibilities. This extra time you will gain is for you and your family to spend together or separately as you wish, for all of you need your own space to develop your own interests. Again, do not listen to the ego, for you are in this world and in this life to learn and develop your abilities and senses.

This change can come for you since you want it so much, but the other way is to be ill eventually and unable to do anything you want. There is really only one choice! Take your time with this process and do not try to do it all at once.

What you can do first is your list of what work you do through each week. This is about finding where your problems are.

Then secondly, find what you can delegate fairly to others by way of family interaction or paying someone to help. This is the delegation of excess duties that take up your time and cause stress.

The third one on your way back to a good balanced life is to spend this special time that you have made by doing what you enjoy. Spend some of it with your family but do keep some time for yourself by doing whatever makes you happy. This is your reward for achieving a better balance in your busy life.

Do not forget to ask for help from God and your angels so you can start this process and continue through with it. Only accept your inner Spirit's words and turn away from your ego, for it will continue to make you seek the gratification of being indispensable. This is a downward path, and you want to be on the Path towards enlightenment.

With enlightenment, you will feel love for yourself and you will find it is wonderful. Life is going forward, so my friends start to reorganize your life and move forward into the Light.

I am,
Merlin

ARGON 7/3/12

Dear friends, I wish to tell you the story of the nice people of the world for they seem to be overlooked in the world's environment today.

To be a nice person is not always a compliment to the person labeled so, for it gives forth an image of weakness by not standing up for their rights. A nice person can be spoken of, and seen as a mild and meek character who is unable to do anything but float along with the world. They do not make the running to achieve much in life but appear to be happy enough any way. They seem to be different to others around them and may appear to have a poor self concept. We are here to say that this is not so!

Meek and mild is good, for God said that, "The meek shall inherit the earth," and so it is dear friends.

You have the wrong idea about these people who appear not willing to fight for what they want, for they are usually advanced souls with very strong characters who will turn the other cheek to those who fight for what they want. These mild souls are not of a materialistic nature and they know that there is more to life than taking what they want. They are of a much deeper nature and see that what they have in their life is a gift, and if they receive more, this is a true blessing. They are full of contentment with most areas of their life, but they do feel a difference from others and their way of living. They know that they are different and often they do wonder why this is so. This is an area in which some may feel uneasy. All on earth should aim for a positive part in their makeup, for this is one of the last lessons that life on this earth teaches you. Love of your self is a positive way to see your own self concept and it is a part of love that God wants to see from you. Love is what the world's lessons are all about, and those of you who are advanced need to respect yourself, your way of living and interacting with those around you. Yes dear friends, the mild and the meek are very advanced souls who are in, or nearly at their last life on earth. They radiate calm from within, and once they understand that they are not wrong by being different in the world, they know that this love for themselves is developing them spiritually.

We are sure that you have seen many examples of self love that are not acceptable, such as when people are so full of their own abilities and what they have, and how they can rule others. This type of soul is being dominated by their ego and is still far from learning life's lessons of self restraint and love for others. Yes, they may be seen to have it all and no one will stand up to them, but they are short on God's requirement of care for others around them. They are failing in this lesson of respect and care for others, and what they feel for themselves is not selfless love but a domination of others. They still have much to learn and will do so one day.

When it comes to being finally taken back to be with God your Father, you need to be living similarly to the way that they are in Heaven. The Lord's Prayer says that, "As it is in Heaven, so will it be on earth". This is not an issue for those who are between lives because they are still learning and growing into the awareness of their Spirit. It is can be an issue for those ruled by their ego and without an open awareness of the perfection for which they should be striving, for they will again be sent of their own free will back for another life to continue to learn and to refine their skills and abilities.

Look around and see if you have any of these meek souls around you. Are there any that seem to take pleasure in living a life similar to that of a child? Remember, if you have seen a young child with its first sight of rain, or snow, or the sea, and have seen them interacting with the elements that are all around them, you will recall the wonder and pure joy that abounds in them and around them. They radiate such a purity of being that comes from deep within their soul, and it is delightful watching this small child. Compare this action of the child to your own reaction to a beautiful view that you have seen before. Do you still gaze with wonder and awe at the sight you see, or do you turn away to other tasks happening at this time? Even with a new view available, do you look quickly and then look away without taking in the wonderful sight that is God's earth. Then it would appear that the simplicity and love of God's world is not strong in you yet, and you are not reacting as an innocent child would.

Now that you are aware of the nature that you have in your journey here on earth, it is up to you to change your attitude and appreciate the gifts that God has given, here on this earth that He made for you. You will find this an interesting prospect if you are close to discovering the child in you.

If you are able to see the lesson in this writing, then you are able to do something about it since you have the free will for this. As with all you do on earth, you are not alone and can ask for heavenly help to achieve the result that you want. It is not a greedy thing, to want to be travelling Home to God, but it is a sign that awareness is growing within you and a change is on the way.

The angels and God Himself are there for you and will help with all you could want to achieve in the life that you want. That way is the way of a child with fresh eyes, who sees all with love and joy in their heart.

Blessings my dear friends,
Argon

MAITREYA 8/3/12

Dear friends, we are together once more for your benefit, for this is the aim of our work for you. We wish to make your journey easier for you and to let you know that life is not always a struggle, but in fact it should be a joy to live your life.

Let us start this discussion with a method that can be used to gain opportunities to give yourself an easier way, so that you may enjoy and flourish in this world that you sought to come back to. You have come back to learn new lessons or to refine those that you learnt in your last life. It was your free will that chose this particular time, but you took advantage of having experienced the advice of the angels from the higher realm. It is these ideas and thoughts that you wish to utilize on earth this time. You realize that there are many souls who are well on in their journey, and yet, they too have come back to aid the world at this time when all are needed to boost the world's vibrations to help the New Age to come in. Without extra help it would be a difficult task while the world is in the state it finds itself in now. Perhaps you may be one of these dear devoted souls who have returned to do all you can to help the world return to stability. While you live on earth, regardless of your stage of development, you will continue to learn lessons, for perfection is what you aim for, but only in Heaven is perfection found.

We of the heavenly realm want you to really enjoy this life due to your consent to return to this life to help. You may not remember why you are on earth now, but you will feel a deep compulsion to achieve and you will intuitively know what you are doing. In the mean time, you can still enjoy yourself. You will be in touch with your inner self and will know or learn that the Law of Manifestation is your way of accessing what you would like to have. Your life can be full of truly great experiences and you can show your advanced skills to others by modeling or teaching. When you have the abilities that you do, you will find that like attracts like, and many of your friends, or those you meet will be of similar mind. What a wonderful way of increasing the outpouring of love for God and His earth. This as we have already shown, is the way to help the world and give it the positive vibrations that are needed.

You have heard of the word karma also, and simplified this means, "What you sow, so shall you reap". This is what we are returning to you, for you have given yourself so selflessly that this will be repaid with what you pray for to make your life easier and more fun. Many of you will be past wanting the material gains of others and so what could make you happier? You are on the Path that gives you a self respect that is required, for this equates to love for yourself which replicates Gods love for you, His child. You can still like a nice home and furnishings, and this is not to be ashamed of, for anything that you have and get are gifts from God. Do not feel that to have objects you like around you are a sign of the ego taking back the power that it has lost, for you know this is not so. Creative works are a wonderful way of self expression and can be thoroughly enjoyed while you are fulfilling your duty. Duty is not a chore of mindless hard work, but it is part of the wonderful whole picture of your life, for you need the balance to keep yourself on track.

How does one get to the stream of manifestation? This is a question that many ask and rightly so. This is your way of gaining what you want and not everyone knows the secret. It should not be a secret but there are those who try and do not quite get the recipe right, and so we will try to explain to you. When in meditation, you find that your mind is stilled and you become part of the great intuitive Universal Mind where all happens as needed. It is like going to a shop. You need to go to the right place, ask for what you want and then wait for it to arrive. We are presuming that this is an order store for this example. If your order does not arrive, you will go back to the store and ask what the problem is and perhaps find that the description you have given was not totally apt and your order was not able to be sent. This is when you stop and think deeply about what you really want and then give a very close description so that there can be no mix up. The same idea goes when asking for what you want. Wait until you are very sure, and if you do not have a name for what you want, then give a very accurate description. Be sure or you may get something very different to what you are presuming you are asking for. If finances are needed, then decide what you want to buy or do with the money. The final move in manifesting is to remember that God's wealth needs to be spread around, otherwise the supply will stop. When you share and give, you are demonstrating your love for others and this then may be a part of fulfilling their desires.

It is an interwoven area, and once you find the way, you will be rich beyond belief, and not just financially, as the greed in you will not exist. Instead you will be part of the world that continues to give love, for you will believe that all that in God's world can be yours, and you will then give the same with love to others who need.

You are a part of the Universal Mind!

This is your reward for following the great Universal Mind which is available to all who seek it. You are among the very blessed at this time, so use this information wisely and you will gain God's Kingdom here on earth, as it is written in the Bible.

I am,
Maitreya

KRISHNA 9/3/12

Today is a wonderful day for you, for you are in a world that is slowly turning away from the old ways and embracing the new style of life that is destined to be available to all on earth. At the moment it is there for you who are aware of the nature of life, and the way of growing through your lives until you reach this level. At this time, there are many who have volunteered to return to this earthly life so that they may be instrumental in helping the process that the world finds itself in. The way has been enriched by these many advanced souls who have offered to give of themselves to this great task. Look around and see the spread of the Word of God! No not in the old way of preaching right and wrong, but in the way of the unseen world of God being accessed so that others may see that life has so much more to offer than it was thought before.

The knowledge that you can personally alter what is happening in your life, and can ask for the world to give you whatever you wish to make your life happier, or easier, is coming to the forefront of common knowledge. This information is being spread by the media of all types and by those who have psychic abilities and show them. Always there is a problem of this ability being used for financial greed, but due to your raised awareness, there is your own guide inside you that will make you feel uneasy if you feel that you are being misled by the egocentric people.

Stand firm against these who found a kernel of the Truth and used it to grow their own truth.

With this new world, there is already a feeling of lightness and anticipation of what is to come into being. Your spiritual self is coming forward and will guide you, if you let it do so. Besides this, you know that the angels who have been with you since your first life are waiting for you to ask them to help. Without them, your world and life will be less than it could be. It is commonly spoken of but please know that you can ask for a trial request. Of course, do not expect an instant answer but give some time for your request to be manifested. Know too, that when you believe, the process is enhanced and this is a good way of helping it happen. If you believe, then you will find that all manner of wishes can come true! Start with a small request such as a sign from your angels and start to look at all that enters your life, such as number codes, perfumes, and white feathers or small coins. Music is another way of contacting you, for if you hear a song play more than once, it may just be a message for you to take seriously. Do not feel ashamed to ask for proof, for it is quite a common ask for those who are just finding this extra dimension in their life. Once it is an accepted fact in your life then you can take it so much further, for you know that you are never alone and that you are always supported by your spiritual helpers. At this stage, many will say to them self that if this can reach me as proof, then what more can be achieved?

Anything you want can happen if only you have the right motivation.

If your request is based on love for those around you and you wish to help them enjoy their life too, choose what is in your heart. There are a few problems that you will face, and they are that if in asking for an item, it will be is used to dominate another then you will not have that object with you for long. If your request is not love based, then it is a greed based premise and not acceptable. If you receive and buy others' services then you are spreading your wealth around, for it is interaction and cooperation that turns the world financially and gives livelihoods to others seeking to provide for their families.

Have you heard the saying, "What goes round, comes around?" It is often used in karma but this time there is an extra meaning for it. When you shop or hire others to do a service for you, you are spreading your finances around to keep the world functioning, but without this sharing, those dependent upon earning money will have a difficult time. When you ask for a gift from the heavenly angels and from God, you are putting yourself into a contract to pass on any benefits that you have gained to others, and this may be an answer to their prayers for manifestation into their life.

The chain of interaction goes a very long way and touches everyone in its cycle. Happiness is the end result of such interactions even when those receiving are not aware of what occurred before they benefitted. The way to use this gift is to give and then you will receive. If you take with both hands for your own benefit, you will not be considered able to handle these great gifts gained by manifesting. This will show that you are not advanced enough in life's learning. You will not be discarded by your God and your angel helpers, but they will wisely wait for you to understand the reasons behind manifestation. They will still be there for you even if it takes more lives for you to live, but your lessons may be given more prominence so that you will not make the same mistake again.

God and His Heaven give love to all who are on earth regardless of the level of behaviour shown by any individual. You just need to understand that at any time you trip and fall, you are helped up and watched with loving care by God and your angels. God is your Father in Heaven and as such, He loves you the way a good human father does his children. Parents help their children to develop, learn and grow into an honest loving people and this is just as it is in Heaven.

Love to you all,
For I am,
Krishna

ORAGON 13/3/12

This is a way to illustrate to you that there is more to what you seek than you could realize.

We are going to give to you some examples of what is coming for the advanced ones who are nearly Home. We will start with the idea that you will all be of the angelic type and sit around on clouds playing harps. This of course is an embellished idea from the early days of religious paintings. We are sure that you know that this could not be the case, but it does sound good! So to show you how your continuing life of learning will proceed after your final life on earth, we will give you some ideas.

You know that in your lives you have been developing skills that can continue from life to life. You will find that the same interests will follow you through to the next lives that you have, though, you may go into trying a different area of serving mankind once you arrive. This can be totally new for you and it is usually quite rare, for usually you have had in mind what it is you want to do to serve. Most of you will have certain interests that you regard as important to your life and to others. To begin with, you will find that you will be given space to find your way about the heavenly realm. This will not take much time, for you are all ready familiar with this due to the time spent there between your lives from the past. You will be given time to rest and visit with your loved ones who greeted you as you arrived in the Light. You will find that you will be different to the person you were on earth, for you may have been aged, sick, or in an accident when you finally came to Heaven.

Life is like it is in Heaven, but Heaven vibrates at a much higher rate, and so, as familiar as it is, it will appear fresher and brighter and full of the love of each person for the others around.

There is no money to buy what you would like, for you have found that bottomless well of supply that you were looking for on earth, for then it was called seeking manifestation for all that you wanted in your life and praying for it to arrive. You may choose to have the home you want, or not. You may find that there is little need to rest any more, and you can see great concerts, art works, or indulge in the magnificent gardens.

You see that earth is a poor replica of Heaven. What is done in Heaven will find its way to earth as an idea for others to invent, but you can see the original since it is with us. The joy that you will feel, will continually lift your spirits and cause great amazement until you become used to the wonders that are kept here for you. By getting used to, we do not mean that you will ever tire of such beauty, but you will be able to access to whatever you want to see or do. What a heavenly idea, don't you think?

Your work will not seem like the work on earth, for when you toiled, your experiences were often boring, difficult, dirty or dangerous. This is the way of many stressful jobs on earth. You will do that which you enjoy serving mankind, but at the same time your learning continues on this plane of life. You will never stop learning for your Spirit will never die, and so you continue with this inbuilt desire to move forward to the next level of your experience. There is not just one level for you to stay in, for remember that God told of His Home having many rooms, and He was referring to all the different areas that you will go to as you travel on your journey onward. You will continue to live in your Spirit as it carries you further on.

What will you look like, you ask? Well you are a being of Light and as such, you continue to exude this Light out ward to others. Those who are in the interim of earth lives can stay the way they looked in their last life, and they will be seen by those who knew them as they did at their prime of life. They can wear the clothes they liked on earth or they can change to their idea of angel robes. It sometimes is not thought of and the being is just as they are, a soul of Light. What appears to be for some is due to their misconceptions or learning on the human plane, and their life will be what they considered it should to be after their "death". They will return to a new life when it is time and they will know what this will be like, but as with most, except as very young children who accept all that they see, they will not recall this time in between. This memory may come later if they are an advanced person who is gaining an understanding of love and a loving God in their time. As you probably know, this is the sign is of feeling that there is more to life, and feeling unsettled and searching to find out what this could be. It is at this time that one usually finds God and their guardian angels, and this then leads them to finding their Spirit which is inside all those who live on earth.

When life is based on advancing your learning it will change for the better, and wondrous things will happen for you. On arriving in Heaven for the last time, you will be overjoyed at seeing your family and friends and at seeing the new life and the surrounds that are now for you to enjoy. There are so many jobs available for you to choose from and incorporate the skills and interests that you had during all of your lives. Look forward dear friends, for the saying that "The world is your oyster", is so true!

This is what is to come for you, this and so much more! This is merely an introduction to your future time in Heaven, and there is much to look forward to in all the other rooms in God's Home. Enjoy the thought and your vibrations will rise in expectation of the love and the way that is yours. More is to come! What a wondrous idea all this is, and it will be yours and everyone else's eventually.

You never die but will live for an eternity. Forever!

This is God's promise to all of you.

I am,
Oragon

KRISHNA 14/3/12

We are going to speak of the time that is about to go into history and this way was not good for living the life of God.

Of course we are talking about this era that is finalizing itself as the New Age comes into existence. It has not been a very God like experience, for if you look around you will find that there are many who did not obey His Commandments. These Commandments are similar to those in different religions, for within many religions and beliefs of the world, there are very similar writings and beliefs that have come down through the ages. The story of a great flood is one known to nearly all in the world and it has come down through the ages in very similar detail. If you take a few different religions and read about their beliefs, you will find an amazing coincidence between their stories, their way of life and beliefs, and yours.

That the world has not followed the rules set out to live by is distressing for we heavenly ones who are trying to help you grow towards your Spirit, and you are very much the poorer for this. This is the reason that there is mayhem on earth in so many places. Not just in the war stricken areas but in the community places that call them self democratically minded, and in advanced conditions. There are those who seek to rule others with threats and violence as well as the persons who want to dominate in their own home and families. Your home is a sacred area that one should give blessings for, for your family is a gift to you and is part of you. You do not own these special persons in your life.

No-one owns another person!

This is the way it should be, and these relationships should be based on love. There is not enough love in the world at this time, and the New Age is all about love for your fellow man and love of God's world. There is a lack of ease around and by this we mean that there is a feeling of insecurity throughout the countries, and this negativity is helping those who are of a dominating nature. Look at all the illness in the world. There are diseases that are growing stronger and sicknesses are difficult to cure. More and more strange diseases are showing up and the medical world is struggling to keep up with finding cures.

If we followed God's rules, this poor standard of health would not be taking over. The egotistical who want to rule all they see, would not be gaining power from others who are indeed fearful of the world as it is now. The news is hard to ignore, for with modern technology you all have access to what is occurring in the world, virtually as it is happening. It is hard to ignore all that is without being pessimistic about the future of life of this world. It is why many are saying that the end of the world is coming. It is not, but the world does need a great deal of help for it to turn itself about and thus gain positive vibrations.

Turning what is, into the opposite side of force will not be easy, but it can be done. That is why many advanced souls are being born. The number being born into the world at the moment is the greatest it has ever been before, and so to help the world, these souls have the mandate to help all who need it. These persons are not going to take over the world as the past has seen of different races, but they are going to infuse their positive vibrations throughout, where ever they go.

Infusing positive energy into your life is really very easy, and so you too can become part of the great solution to the future of this world. Firstly, you need love for the people of this earth, and love for the world that God made for you to live in. Look about, for indeed it is a wondrous place to live. Through the media you can see the wars and the bad happenings, but also, you will see the wonders of this place you call home. Focus on the bright, the colourful, the wonderful sights, and all the different features that make up this huge globe that you live on. You can see the places that are above you, around you, and below where you live are able to lift your thoughts into a higher level and make you want to protect what you all have. This then forms you into a group, and although we know that peer pressure can have some difficult results, it can also be a strong force for the good of a group and whatever their focus is.

As always, there is the power of prayer, for these souls who are returning are well aware of their purpose in this life and will be able to pray with the right intensity to cause the vibrations to gain strength. Meditation is on the increase, for it not only helps the ones who meditate but also those interact with them. This is a sign! The ways of the New Age people are gaining strength and they are using their ability to bring heavenly helpers into the equation. In the past, there was little known about the way of the so called psychics and they were dispelled as charlatans, but now, more and more are finding that they too have these abilities.

All on earth have these so called psychic abilities, and for those who have discovered theirs, it is the awakening of the Spirit within their soul.

You have heard that only a small part of your brain is being used, so think what you will be capable off when you learn to use it fully. The New Age will be known more fully when your mind and brain are fully utilized, and this is not far away.

The first step then is to go back to obeying God's Laws as given to you as a guide to living a good life. Then you can send an out pouring of love to your heavenly Father, which will bring good vibrations into dominance in the world arena. With this awareness of God in your life you will be able send prayers of love to those who are lost in the darkness of this world. This is the way forward; forward to help bring in this wonderful New Age which is prophesied so all can live in the richness of God's love.

Dear friends, it is for you to take the lead and show and tell of the wonders that can come. The people of the world will see that the rebels' domination of the world is not the way of God.

I am,
Krishna

ORCHUN 16/3/12

Now is the time to speak of the way of your life.

Is it a good way do you think? Is it just an existence since you are not interested in what you do? Do you not have friends, time, or hobbies? This then is not a successful life and it needs to change, for you were not sent to earth to live such a life. Life should be full of pleasurable activities, of laughter, friends and love. You may have this in your life, but also on another level you can be stressed from not getting out of this life what you feel you should. This would be seen to be a false way of interacting with life, for if you are acting a role of enjoying yourself at times, then you need to change. These two examples are equally not right for anyone.

Look at the way that you should be living. As you look around, you will see many who radiate happiness and joy. They too have time deadlines and many of the same problems that you do too, but they are handling it a lot better. How do they do it? Watch and see. They pay attention to the moment, and do not waste their energy on going over their planning of what is to be happening later in the day, or the week, or the month.

They do not focus on the future.

They take in hand what is happening in the Now of their time.

They too can feel stress or pain like so many others, but they have a naturally happy outlook and this is why they enjoy their time. They do not allow their problems to take over their time. If you are not a natural bubbly personality, do not worry, for you can find your own way to your happiness. It needs a little bit of confidence and a promise to yourself to think of the moment that you live in, and then see what you can enjoy in your situation. It may be that you work around others who are not so happy or those who are too busy organizing for much later in time in life. Even knowing that this time may not come will still cause them stress, and then give out a real feeling of negative vibrations to affect you.

There is only Now in your life. Each split second is what you are living. Yes, if you are in business you do need to plan for the future, but you need to find one who you trust implicitly and delegate to them. Share the problem and brainstorm, and then you will be able to get back to enjoying your surroundings. If you only have bare walls to look at, then put up a picture of your family, or one of a sight you like, or place some flowers in your area. Fresh flowers are a wonderful way of influencing the environment and since they are living breathing parts of the outside world, they have the ability to bring in fresher air and positive feelings to whoever is around. Think of all the colours that are flowers. Do you have a favourite flower or pot plant? Some plants can grow inside and this too will help you feel more at ease.

If you dislike your job, then you will need to look harder to make your surroundings more comfortable and to provide your mind with the ease that it needs to function without stress. Alternatively you can look elsewhere for work but don't let this need overcome you. It will happen if you take time to visualize yourself working in a different and happier area. Don't forget your angels and the help they are always ready to give. Just ask!

What you need to do is to find what you enjoy being around and bring it into your work world, for a change is what is needed to revive you. Everyone has to do some type of work, so if others can enjoy themselves while earning their living, you can too. Change, along with delegation within a team frame work is what can lead to better work skills, and changing the environment to introduce that which you enjoy and love around you, is a great start to this new attitude of yours.

When others notice the change in you, do not shrug it off with embarrassment but thank them, for it is proof that you have succeeded in helping yourself to a better balanced life. Share your secret with those who ask how this miraculous change happened, for they too may be feeling too much of the stress of life. If you find you are falling back to your old ways, then stop and reorganize what is around you, for it is said that a change is as good as a holiday.

You can make a difference in your own world and help others too, but you need to start living in the Now of your life, for stress comes from trying to prepare for the future that we don't know, because it is still coming.

Do it my friends, and you will be amazed at how much you can enjoy the mundane parts of life, for even here in your daily life you can find beauty in it. There is beauty all around you that you can use to bring the Light and grace into where you spend a lot of time.

I am,
Orchun

MERLIN 17/3/12

We, the angelic support for all on earth, are here for you at all times.

So many of you know that we are in your life, but some do not and we can help them live the life that they want if only they would open the way. We are not here to direct your life but to give when asked. The word "give" covers a lot of areas including material supply, as well as spiritual support. We cannot give until we are asked but we watch and see the turmoil in your life. This rule of your own self choice is one of the necessary rules that we obey, for this life of yours is to help you grow. You grow through the interaction of your thoughts and with what you do as you live each life here on earth. This earth is a large school but it need not be a difficult one. It has been said that sorrow and struggling are the way you learn your lessons best, but this does not need to be when you are of an advanced nature, although there are some who can learn through making mistakes. They do this by being aware of the nature of man and the way that they live, and they will then feel that they are doing something wrong and change it for comforts' sake. In a major trauma, it becomes very difficult for those who are less advanced to see their way through the stress in their mind, and so this becomes a difficult and almost impossible task. They do not have the ability to put that which has happened to them down to karma or ego.

Throughout your thousands of lives, you have been with the same groups at different times and therefore gained some good and bad karma from these relationships. If you have not found a way to interact with one or more of these souls to find a solution, you will be put in a similar situation until the lesson is learned and the karma satisfied. Perfection is not demanded in these interactions, for that can only occur in Heaven, but it needs to be seen that the lessons learned have given you the ability to work out what has gone before. We will state again that perfection happens to only the most developed Spirits in Heaven. Once you ascend to Heaven, you will find you are still aiming for perfection with all the lessons that occur in the many "rooms" in God's Home. This happens until you find your final eternity of your Spirit, which is, my dear friends, a long way off. We ask that you do the very best you can in life and do it with love and acceptance of others' ways. It is known by you who are near your last earthly life that love is the basis of all, and until you show this to your fellow man, the world will not be as it should.

Tolerance is based on love. The world needs this tolerance.

There are many people that you do not accept for their way of life and attitudes. You do not have to give love as you do to your friends, but just be aware that they are not as advanced as you and give prayers and blessings to support them. This may not seem much of a help, but once you bring in the angelic realm through these prayers it opens the way for help to be given to the situation around them. They are not stripped of their free will, but the situation around them can be changed to give them the chance to use their free will to change themselves positively. This is the way of the future, for as we have said, there are many now who have been born especially to pray and do all they can to help this world move into the New Age. The free will of these souls chose to come back and do this work for the betterment of the world as it is at this point. You are a part of this movement.

Tell others of what you have found in these writings and you will be helping some who may not have been able to discover the Truth of Life. They may be able to take some comfort from you about their life and what it entails, and this is giving you a karma that makes your life a happier place. Your life of love promotes good karma, and by gaining this, it is a way of learning so much more. You ask how, and we will tell you that it is easier to learn in a calm conducive atmosphere than one of stress. Help others to learn this especially if they are in the depths of despair for it may not help them now, but you will have sown the seed, and the soil it is in may just be fertile enough to start growing. Imagine if many of you dear readers do this as a way to serve your fellow man, what a great service you are doing. The Now of your life and theirs becomes intertwined, and the message of angelic help is available for all those who feel out of control of their life. You will become a teacher and guide for many to reach out to gain what you have, and then they too will grow to be in the same position to guide those close to them.

The wheel that you start rolling will gather momentum, and you will be doing your best with love in your soul for those around you in your life.

I am,
Merlin

MAITREYA 18/3/12

Welcome dear friends, for we are writing these items for the benefit of all of you who are actively seeking the Truth in your life.

We wish to discuss what seems to be a common problem in your life, for you are not alone in seeking your way Home. There are so very many who are very close to finding the Truth that illustrates what life is all about, or should be about. This is due to the influx of well advanced souls who are here to do what they can to bring in the New Age which is upon us. The state of the world needs some help, and sooner rather than later. Many, who were residing in Heaven after their last life, have volunteered to be a part of this group who would help the world rid itself of the negative life styles that are abounding. The negative in today's life, even in the advanced countries, is not a way to bring in the splendour of what is coming. The focus for those involved in this life of evil is on themselves as grasping people, for they want to take all the power they can for themselves. They wish to be the dominant force and rule as much of the world as they can. Of course you know that this is why the fighting in the world is occurring now and the power to control others has always been the main reason for countries to fight.

We shall now tell you what needs to be for those of you who are on the verge of awakening, and this is the way you can help your world. We have touched on this a few times in these writings but the whole way of using your abilities is still a little vague in your minds. This is known, for we watch all of you, and there is still a little wariness that sending positive vibrations it is not sufficient. You all believe in the power of prayer, but the way of raising this large world's vibrations is seen as too big a miracle.

Let us begin to explain for you. You find that praying is a positive force, but that it does not seem enough when dealing with such an enormous task as taking the world from one end of the vibration pendulum to the other. So you see that you are looking at the problem from a much smaller view, and this is the human view formed by your limited abilities. When you begin to look at the problem from the heavenly view, that God did create this earth for you and is mighty, then you can see that when you give prayers you do help to save the world and to guide all who live on earth. He can take these prayers and use them in a monumental way of which you could not understand.

This is the eye of your problem and you need to forgo your view point of how this may work and take on the higher premise that all is possible. God is telling you that this is so and your faith is rewarded when you ask Him to help. He cannot interfere with the lives of any on earth at this time or ever, since His promise of giving you free will, stops Him. This is where you come into the story, for when you pray for help and the betterment of the world, then He can then step in and do His miracles. Do you see that by praying for the souls of the world to have a better life, you are doing what God is not able to do until you ask Him?

God needs you just as you need God in this life.

Without this help, the future is looking dim. Look only at the Now of time, for if the ways of the world are not attended to Now then it will be difficult, if not impossible to stop the world from travelling along this track that it is on.

This is what the New Age is about! It is a prophecy of hope for the future, and we all know that prophecies are not always fulfilled without turning the mind to it and preparing the way. It is similar to planting a vegetable garden, for you need to set the soil to right and then sort out what would grow best, and then you care for the plants, for without constant care they would likely die or not give a good crop.

You are setting the first steps in process by praying for God to help and in this way you are sending Him good vibrations to work with, for this is a part of your prayers in blessing those who are in a difficult way of life. By continuing to pray for a basis in which the New Age can flourish, you are providing the continuing conditions needed by God and His many, many angelic helpers to improve the world at this dire time.

This is the job that you accepted between your last life and this one, when you were shown what you could do to serve mankind. Many of you know that you have a special role on earth but are not sure of what it could be. Since you are reading our words, you are aware of your role from the writings within and will now start to do your special work. We bless you for your help, for as you are helping us, we are also helping you. You are not alone in your dedication, and constant dedication is what we need from you and all who are involved in setting the way clear for this New Age.

You are doing this for the world and for all your descendants, and know that you have been given a better explanation so that you will do a wonderful job. Where there is understanding, the processes involved are much easier for you to continue daily. Again, we send our blessings to you, dear friends.

I am,
Maitreya

MERLIN 19/3/12

Welcome to this story, for it is coming to you straight from the heart of all that is. We are going to tell you about what you are coming from and to where you are going.

Since you have been reading the stories before this, then you know what an important job you have to do! We will start with the past, for as you know from these readings, there is much to learn from what happened before. It is a guide to what could happen in the future if the setting is similar. This age today has so much more than before and so we will need to take the situation of Now and that which has passed, into consideration. We are of course talking about your life story, and how you are involved with all that happens in this world of yours. How can this be related to the past you ask? Well, if you look at the way in which past generations have lived and the conditions that they had, you may just gain and inkling of what we mean. In the past eras, there was great poverty and great wealth living side by side, and this was not that long ago. Look at today's world and there is a distinct increase in the standards of life. The rich and well off are becoming richer, for they have the power and use it to their own advantage. The poorer are kept busy by trying to survive financially and are struggling for their existence. This becomes a problem for balancing the two levels together, for though there are some who take the cause of the less strong, they too are unable to do much and have little impact on the situation.

Let's look at how this was solved in the past, for we do know that there has been and will be, and this is that the very poor and the less advanced who will always struggle. This may be a part of their karma from a previous life, so keep this in mind regarding the result. What happened slowly was the joining of these people together so they had more impact on any problem they found was affecting their lives. The more who joined in, the stronger they became, and this lasted until a short time ago when the wealthier felt threatened by this growing force. As well, there was growing together of the middle class who feel that they too rule the work ethos with the wealthier, and they also set about to diminish the power of the workers. Of course we are talking about the Union of workers who have in many ways sabotaged their own power by making demands that were not rational. We are sure that you have all heard about the demands made for a large mark up of wages without the extra work to go with it. This has caused a ridicule of these organizations and they truly have deserved this. If the members had been more aware of the type of people who stood for the positions in the Union movement, they would have been more careful when electing them. Many of these persons are of the idea that they are superior to those they support, or they gain a different view of what should be once they are instilled in their office. This does not refer to all of those leading the Union of workers, but enough are like this, and the less radical Union leaders find that the ridicule rubs off on them and the workers too. Now you find that the Unions have had a lot of their power taken away. With this, you will find that those who do not support the Union are given the same conditions that the Union gains for their members. Why should they support this movement financially since they are given the benefits any way? This is why the movement now has less members, and this is the why the Unions are weaker and cannot stand against those who rule the industries.

Let's look back at history when the movement started and see how miners for example, handled the situation. They were totally united and would support each other regardless of the financial and personal cost. They stood shoulder to shoulder and all shared whatever they had just to survive.

This was togetherness that showed the strength of uniting and working together as one.

The leaders within the movement they did not try to rise above the other workers, but they were able to give their thoughts for the management of unfair situation to help others who were less able.

Today there is a need to balance the wealth and power, but it will be difficult for these souls in control to let go of this strength they enjoy. The feeling of discontent will grow and workers will think back to when they had proper representation and how this gave them pride in themselves and their jobs. We foresee a change coming, indeed it has started, and it will be part of the New Age. This time will be for sharing, respect, and love for all in the world. People will again band together to gain the positive vibrations necessary to turn around that which is unfair.

History is talking to you and the future is in your hands. Use this example for the betterment of all you who live, work and interact on this earth. Start now but keep the peace, for this too is a lesson from the original fight of the Unions to gain strength and respect. Be a part of what you need to for the future if you wish it to be fair for all.

I am,
Merlin

KRISHNA 21/3/12

Welcome to you dear friends.

This is a time of understanding which is to be a great help in what you do, regardless of what else you are involved in. This is to help you find your way for we do not want you to worry about what it is you are here to do.

Let us start with the idea of giving to others, for you hear from us that this is the way of showing love to those around you. We know that you all want to do the right thing, and with the hints that we give, you should be able to find your way more easily. Here are some ideas for you to try. There are many ways you can help by coming forward with your need to do so. Most people would love some help in the area that they have decided that they can support most, and the area that we are writing about is that of giving alms to the poor. This, you will concede, is a great thing to do, for this can ease their burden greatly.

There are so many in need that you are unable to aid all, so you need to decide what you can afford and which area of need causes a response within you. If you feel a need to care for a child in a poor country, then the benefits would be great as this gift would be passed on for the next generations. The poverty stricken places of the world are desperately in need of education, and once one child is educated, then others will receive the benefits in terms of that person's passing on their expertise.

Then the other choice can be to buy goods such as plumbing goods to enable water to be brought to the villages. With water, you know so much is possible from general cleanliness, hygiene and the treatment of diseases. As well, water can be used to grow their food thus allaying the starvation that many areas have. These all intertwine and support each other, so the idea of supporting in this way has enormous rewards.

The other ways that you can support those seeking help is to look closer to home. Since you live in relative wealth, such as you have more that those who are destitute and the poor of other countries, you do have more than the basic needs to live a good life. Even so, there are still costs, and so you do have to look at your own finances as a guide to the amount of help that you can give. There are very many who seek help for medical research as well as other medical areas. There are also many in your own back yard who are in need of help such as the elderly on a basic income and who need someone to help them in their home, and children in dire need of protection, animals also needing care, and the environment. There are so many other areas that are calling for recognition that there are too many to note, but of course you cannot do what you would like to help them all.

The solution is to choose which area is closest to your heart and then decide how many of these organizations you can help. You are showing your love regardless of what plea you are responding to. You will have a positive impact and that is all you can do, unless you are very wealthy and if this is so we hope that this is a consideration in what, and how many you support. As long as you give with love whatever you can do or afford, you are achieving the aim of helping and supporting your fellow man. This is all you can do financially, but what about spiritually?

Bring the power of your prayer to your wanting to help, and the process is magnified.

With this request for help from God and His angels, God can then intercede for the benefit of those who are prayed for. Your help is then enhanced and taken to a higher level, and at this level miracles can and will happen. This is a lead into the New Age that is beginning, where love and care for your fellow man will be paramount in all who live.

When you do what you can for them, no more is expected from you, and you can rest easy that you are living for your fellow man. We bless you for this that you do for others.

I am,
Krishna

VISHNU 23/3/12

Today dear people, I wish to tell you of the times of worry and stress that can cause a soul to return home earlier than was planned for their life.

We will begin with the way that you cope with all that happens to you during your daily routine. Stress is all around you no matter where you go or how you feel, for it is and always has been a big part of life. This too is a lesson sent to you, for you need to learn how to cope with these situations that you find yourself in. Sadly, there are many who do not cope and decide to remove themselves from this life, for they do not have the mechanisms to work against the problems that they face.

These souls, dear people, are not sent to hell as often indicated by religious associations, but they are gently taken back and helped to find the answer to what their problems were.

They are not shunned by God and His angels but are given a chance to see what they could have done, and they are then prepared to return to a similar situation in their next life.

This life for you is a learning process, and you need to keep returning until your soul is advanced enough to cope when in such a situation again. If you have one in your life who was not able to cope with the pressure, please do not feel horror or blame for them or yourself, for it was only a lesson they tried to learn but were not advanced enough to find the solution. Send your love to them in your prayers and say that you understand. Forgive them, as God forgives them and you, for all your transgressions. Look to a young child who is trying to learn society's rules and also learning to read and write, and you will see that some do not always cope with this. They are too young to know of coping methods and so they need to be taught by one who is sensitive to their needs and the plight that they find themselves in. If you see a very unhappy young child then you will know that they cannot cope with what is happening in their life at that time. They need comfort and help to know what to do, and some of the expectations need to be removed from them to ease their load. This is how it is in Heaven when a soul returns from an unfinished life span with a fear, and always a regret of what they have done. Once they return to Heaven, they know that their problem has not gone away but it is indeed made worse by the knowledge of the hurt they have caused their loved ones. They are received with love and understanding and no blame is attached to what they have done. For you see that all on earth and in Heaven are God's creations. He is the Father to all that is, including you and every one on earth. You are all brothers and sisters, and it is compassion such a relationship needs to be given to all who struggle with life problems.

At any time in your life you will find that there are big problems or small ones and you do not need to fix them by yourself. Listen to your inner voice, your Spirit that lives on through all the lives you will have until you return Home to God Himself. You are never alone, and during the good times you may feel that you are doing it all by yourself, but know that you are being watched with love to see what you are doing. When times are not as good and you feel distressed, do not forget that you have access to help in your time of trouble.

This is when you should bring your memory to the fore and pray to God, for He will send His angels to you, and if you listen to that quiet voice within your heart you will receive the right guidance that you are seeking.

Your problem may not go instantly, but remember that this is a learning time and needs to be experienced, and ideas of how to manage will be promoted. Yes, these ideas come from your spiritual helpers but you will need to implement them. You will never be given the wrong advice by these special helpers. They are there for you as soon as you ask for them. Treat their advice with gratitude and know that nothing can befall you that is in any way wrong for the situation. If you do not feel at ease with your advice then check and see if it could be that part of you, the ego, trying to take back control of you. The control that you have given Him is what the ego had over you for the earliest years of your developmental lives. When you become aware that you are a developed soul who is well on the way to being responsive to your Spirit only, the ego recedes into the background, but not without some last attempts at ruling you. It will give you the most inept instructions to try to hold onto you, for when you are distressed you are unable to think clearly and be very sure of hearing the voice of your Spirit guiding you. Be aware of what you are being instructed to do, for at this stage of your development you know what is right and wrong. If you are unable to hear a voice directing you to good thoughts, then notice your inner feelings, for if you feel unease the information is most likely not coming from the appropriate source.

You will never be punished for making mistakes but you will find yourself again in a similar situation so that you may learn your lesson, and you can then move onto the next stage of your learning. All of life is a lesson, and all souls are having these same lessons as they travel the Path back to Heaven. Use any help that you can find but make sure that it is the right advice, for you do not want to repeat this lesson if you can help it.

Feel love, and direct love and your prayers to those who stumble in a lesson of life. Love for all is what you need to send, for it lifts them to higher states and they will know that they are not criticized for stumbling but are being wished the best you can for them in their journey.

They will return and be prepared for this lesson when it appears to them, and they will be better able to learn the necessary problem solving skills.

I am,
Vishnu

ARGON 24/3/12

We are going to speak today about the areas that you seem to have a problem with. Yes there are many, and all different for different souls, but this one seems to be the most common one overall.

Let us begin dear friends, with this statement, and this is that you are struggling with keeping up your good intentions as you find your way through your busy day.

If we say to you that you are not always focused on the journey that you are on, we are sure that you will agree. There is always some problem that arises that will cause you to divert from your good intentions. Let us try to illustrate one of these! When you are driving your car and you are put at risk by another person's dangerous driving, or even a pedestrian stepping of the path, you use profanities that are not normally part of your vocabulary. Immediately you may feel remorse, or even later when the incident comes to mind, and you know that you should not have spoken so, for you are using the Lord's name in vain and this is not what His name is for. We understand that in times of stress it is common to call out His name for this is a call for help from Him. We take this incident as one of those times where you realized what a dangerous situation you found yourself in and called to God as a cry for help. In this way, can you see that this really is not a move against your beliefs? We accept the conditions that it was made in, and if it was a little inappropriate, do not feel that you have gone against your inner guidance.

Now in contrast, let us look at those who use profanities for the sake of gaining personal attention. This is not the way of a righteous person! You will at all times know that this person is not an advanced soul and is still in control of his ego, and of course does not know any better. To these souls you send your blessings, and pray that they will advance into a better way of speaking. This is the only help for these people and it is a good thing you do when you pray for them. God can then become involved with them as you have asked for this help. You may feel annoyed with these people but they are your brothers and sisters, and as such, they deserve the same chance to grow spiritually as you have. Make it a habit to say, "Bless you", to any person you feel pity or anger towards and you are then doing your job well.

We also find that there are situations that you find yourself in, in that they challenge your ability to stay focused on the course that you have discovered,. You will also be aware that it is possible to fall off the Path that you are on and this is a concern for you when in such a situation. Let us look at such a case. If you happen to talk to your working partners in a strong tone of voice, and state that the process will be done your way, even knowing that you are meant to value every one's opinion, you may feel that inner voice speaking to you reminding you of the correct way of dealing with the situation. This will be your Spirit reminding you. Remember though that sometimes you are in a situation that all around you are at odds with each other, and you are in the position to take the leadership role. Do not stress about such an incident, for we understand the ways of the world and that sometimes you need to do this in the situation that you find yourself in. This way may not work successfully but it may be better to try than to stay in a dead lock. As long as this does not become intrinsically part of your way of dealing with problems, then it is accepted for this time. Plan though, for the next time and set in motion ways that will help smooth the way to a better working relationship. What we are trying to show you is that nothing is set rigidly in place, for there are times that need you to take responsibility above all that you do normally. Your beliefs will stay in place, but there is plenty of leeway, as long as you remain aware of God's way of working

When you are ready, you will find within your Spirit a part that will ensure you stay within the boundaries of what is expected for you to continue advancing. Remember that there is no total perfection on earth, even though this is what you are aiming for. Keep your goal in place but be realistic as to what you do, and you will continue on your Path Home to God.

He is a forgiving God, full of love and trust in you. He will not turn away from you if you trip or stumble on your journey.

His hand will be extended to you as you are helped up again and are pointed back to the Path you need to be on. He is full of love for you, His child, and is with you regardless of the times that you stray, and remember that you will end your journey in His home.

Use all that you have learnt on this wondrous trip to guide you onward and trust in your Spirit residing within you. Remember that you have your guardian angels with you at all times and as soon as you call them, they will respond.

This lesson is all about love, trust, and the support of God and His helpers in Heaven. Believe and move forward with confidence, for self confidence is a self love which is a requisite to continue onward. With self love you know that you are spiritually led and are very close to your goal. Keep going and do not stress about the few times that you feel that you are not using the knowledge that you have attained.

Dear friends, I am,
Argon

VISHNU 25/3/12

Let us begin dear friends, with the promise of a wonderful time.

When you ask? Well dear friends, all of your lives, one at a time, should be wonderful for you. God sent you to earth to learn your lessons but He does not want you to struggle, for this is not the best way of learning. In fact this way can turn many against life's lessons and the reasons they are incarnated in this life of theirs. Look at a child in school who is struggling and obviously not happy and you will know that they are unable to learn their lessons well. There is too much stress in their life and stress is the area that causes all other parts of their life to regress into misery.

Being unable to cope is what we understand but we don't know why you do not use your gift of free will to call for help.

Sometimes, we know that the stress is so strong that it is difficult to think and make decisions, but before you reach this level, it is a good idea to write yourself a letter regarding your spiritual life and why you are here.

This letter can be in a formal style, or as notes to remind you of better times so that you can start to remember some of your good times. Make sure you include the love you feel for those around you and how this makes you feel within yourself. Love is what God has for every one of you, for He is Love itself. Write about what you believe and at this stage of your life journey, you will be aware of

God and His angels and that you are not alone. Write in big letters that are well defined stating that,

"God loves me, and I only have to ask for help and He is with me."

When you are feeling the pressures of life, this will remind you that you just need to ask for help and it is yours. Do not dictate what type of help, but just define the problem and ask that it be solved so then you can continue on with your learning. Carry this letter to yourself around with you and use it as a way to cope with your day. Yes, some days can be a struggle, but if you take this problem with you each day, it will continue to grow and fester into a sore. You don't want this to happen, so take the gift that God has given you, and ask for help for anything, even small problems and you will be answered. The angels are interwoven with your life and they are there for all of you and want to help, regardless of the size of your problems. They are able to turn around any situation that you enter and then find unmanageable.

If you do not like to write letters, then you can still give yourself a reminder that can be used in a similar way. Sometimes, you write notes to remind yourself of what you need to buy or where to go, or for numerous other reasons, and here is one way that you can keep your note to the point.

START WITH POSITIVE STATEMENTS:

I am God's child.

I am never alone.

I can ask for help anytime from God and His angels.

My life is happy and stress free.

My problems are being solved.

I am learning life's lessons with love.

There in a nutshell, are your positive statements.

If you wish to make this easier, then photocopy these statements and keep them with you. Do not worry about what you have done wrong, for you will not be judged by God. He will lift you up and help you on your way but,

YOU MUST ASK FOR HELP.

With your right to make your own choices, He and His angels will not interfere with whatever you decide, but pray, talk, or ask Him to help and guide you. Then your life will settle down, as the answers will be provided to solve your problems and show you back to enjoying your life.

Vishnu

A FINAL WORD FROM YOUR ANGEL
WRITERS: 23/4/12

Jan, we thank you for writing our words so that we can share them with so many true believers who are on their Path and helping the world as they go on in this life.

It is a long journey that you are on dear friends, and as such, you are doing such a wonderful job. With the reading of this book, we hope that you have gained the insight to help this world as it travels onwards in the New Age. While you are doing this you are also learning the right way to live your life. This includes how to be aware of the dominating ego's strength, and the positives such as your inner spiritual voice which guides you, and of the help of your angels and guides who are always just a prayer away. God has meant your life to be a wonderful, joyful time. Even the role of karma in your life, both positive and negative is discussed so that you can understand and handle the events that are happening for you.

Use this book, dear friends for it is our way to help you attain your ascension.

Within is a reminder for that which you promised to do before you were born into this life; by praying to God and His angels so that He can help this destructive and negative world learn to love each other so that the glorious New Age can continue to grow.

We send our thanks to you for all you are doing for the NOW of time and for the promised future of the New Age. It is in your hands dear friends, for we are asking you to pray to us so that we may help the world into this wonderful New Age. Without your prayers and asking for our help, we can only watch as the world continues on this destructive path.

Please dear friends, we need very many souls who are aware of helping in this time of Now, for this world is in a difficult dilemma and will not fix itself without all of you and your prayers.

Help!

We need you!

The world needs you!

Your world's brothers and sisters need you!

Only you can to provide a wonderful future for your descendents

It has been our pleasure to show you your way, dear friends.

Blessings and love from,

Merlin, Maitreya, Jesus, St.Germain, Confucious, Serepis Bey, Krishna, and all of your angels writing for this book.

They wish to send their dedication, love and guidance to you.

REFERENCES:

I have used one written reference*. The angels' words are used as my references and I have written their words to the best of my ability. The words or phrases used and emphasized throughout out the writings are those directly given to me by the Ascended Masters. I feel sure that we all have heard some of them, if not all, as well as those referred to from the Bible.

Any mistakes made are due to human error which can enter all work such as this.

I apologize for any that have been unintentionally made.

*Doreen Virtue, Ph.D.
Ascended Masters Oracle Cards.
Hay House, Inc